D0053127

crazy*sexy*
CANCER TIPS

kris carr

FOREWORD BY *sheryl crow*

skirt!

GUILFORD, CONNECTICUT
AN IMPRINT OF THE GLOBE PEQUOT PRESS

To buy books in quantity for corporate use
or incentives, call **(800) 962–0973**
or e-mail **premiums@GlobePequot.com.**

The health information expressed in this book is based solely on the personal experience of the author and is not intended as a medical manual. The information should not be used for diagnosis or treatment, or as a substitute for professional medical care. The author and publisher urge you to consult with your health care provider prior to attempting any treatment on yourself or another individual.

skirt!® is an attitude . . . spirited, independent, outspoken, serious, playful and irreverent, sometimes controversial, always passionate.

Copyright © 2007 by Kris Carr

All rights reserved. No part of this book may be reproduced or transmitted in any form by any means, electronic or mechanical, including photocopying and recording, or by any information storage and retrieval system, except as may be expressly permitted in writing by the publisher. Requests for permission should be sent to skirt!, Attn: Rights and Permissions Department, P.O. Box 480, Guilford, Connecticut 06437.

skirt!® is a registered trademark of Morris Publishing Group, LLC, and is used with express permission.

Contribution from Oni Faida Lampley on pages 120–21 originally published in *Self* magazine, in an article titled, "No More Shame."

Due to limitations of space, photo credits appear on pages 202–3 and constitute an extension of this page.

10 9 8 7 6 5 4 3

Printed in the United States of America

Design by Karla Baker www.typekarla.com

Library of Congress Cataloging-in-Publication Data

Carr, Kris.
Crazy sexy cancer tips / Kris Carr ; foreword by Sheryl Crow.
     p. cm.
ISBN: 978-1-59921-231-9
1. Cancer in women. I. Title.
RC281.W65C374 2007
616.99'40082—dc22
             2007007701

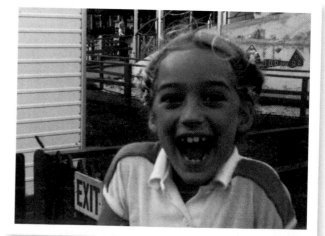

contents

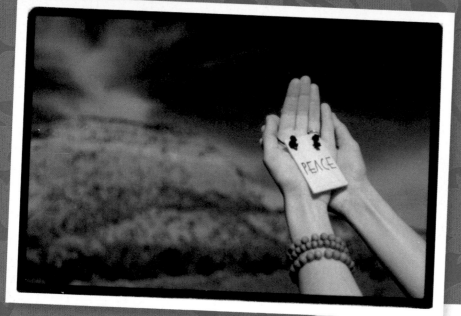

{ dedication }

To my mom, Aura Carr, she taught me
how to be a survivor long before cancer.

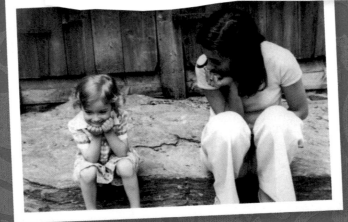

{ foreword } by Sheryl Crow

"Hi, Doug. How are you? Me? Not so great. You know how I'm always calling you to ask you for referrals for newly diagnosed friends? Well . . . this time it's me."

I will never forget the afternoon I received the news I had cancer. The three calls I made first were to my parents, my ex (who happens to be a very well-known cancer survivor), and Doug Ulman, the president of the Lance Armstrong Foundation and a dear friend.

My routine mammogram showed microcalcifications, not unusual for someone my age. It was my ob-gyn who called and said there was no point waiting for six months to check on them, and that a biopsy in both breasts would be wise. It's possible she saved me from having more radical treatment, simply because I didn't wait and instead was diagnosed very early.

Anyone who has ever been diagnosed with a disease will tell you that time stands still in that moment. In fact, it backs up and runs over you on its way past. I barely remember hearing the words "It's cancer," but the tears in my doc's eyes are an everlasting image in my mind.

I called my parents on the way home. My parents are my best friends and have always been there on every level for me. And, in their usual fashion, they calmly alerted my siblings and promptly flew to Los Angeles to be with me. Right behind them were my sisters and my longtime manager, and later, my brother and his family.

Our initiation into Cancer College took place in what felt like a boardroom, with my family and my manager and my oncologist sitting at a very long table looking at visuals of breast ducts, drawings of cells gone wacko, and lots of medical statistics. (I can safely say that my dad is a breast expert now and not by choice.) We learned more about cancer in two hours than I learned about anything in four years of college. The doctor told us that there are many different kinds of cancer and that because mine wasn't in my lymph nodes, I would get off relatively easy. However, the bottom line is, even though the cancer may go away, knowing that you had cancer doesn't. The fear of it coming back doesn't go away, either.

1

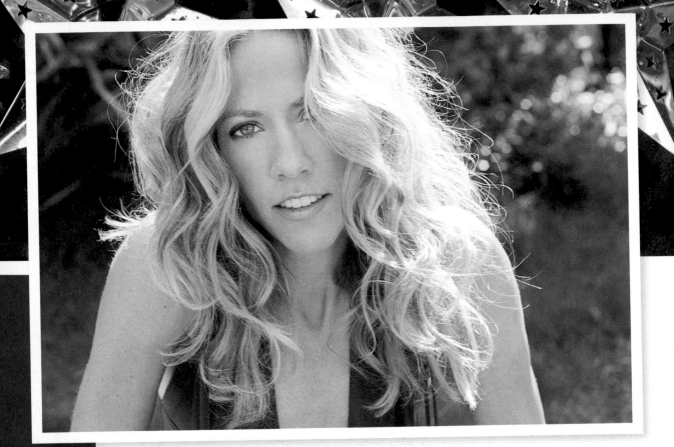

It has been a fascinating journey for me. I have been embraced by an amazing community of women who are survivors or who have lost loved ones to cancer. Women generous in sharing their personal stories. Courageous women who still manage to find humor in even the toughest of circumstances. But the one testimony I believe I heard the most was the correlation of breast cancer to nourishment. My whole life, I have felt like a self-sufficient person, a make-shit-happen kind of gal. Totally fit, healthy eater, meditator for years, that's me. Being diagnosed with cancer really opened my eyes to the fact that anyone can have it and that even though we think we have control over everything in our lives, we don't.

What I was forced to learn, like so many other women I've spoken with, was to put myself first. To really honor myself by saying no to things I don't want to do. This is a very new exercise for me. I have always been a pleaser of the most committed kind. The idea that the breast is very symbolic of nurturing and of nourishment resonates heavily with me because I, like so many other women, have mastered putting everyone else's needs before my own.

For me, the mere act of letting people take care of me was a challenge. It felt completely foreign. The first week of radiation, my mother made eight different kinds of organic soup. My dad got up at the crack of dawn to feed my dogs, make the coffee, pick up the paper. My family took weeklong shifts to take care of me—or just be there. The mere switch to not planning activities, not preparing meals, actually taking naps or just resting, required complete restraint.

Every day since that time, I have reminded myself of what I took from the experience. Things I don't ever want to forget. I look at my breast cancer "tattoos" and am reminded of the expansion that was created in my life because of what I went through and of who I've become, and I am grateful.

There are no real handbooks on what to do first when you get your diagnosis. No one can tell you how the experience is going to go. In my case, I knew I was not going to die, but I also knew, early on, that my life would never feel or look the same. I remember my radiologist saying to me, "Your mission now is to ask yourself every day, 'Am I doing what I want to be doing?'" And I do ask myself that, every day. I try to make the answer yes, even if it requires saying the word *no* and disappointing someone.

My experience was about letting go. It was about really experiencing all that was happening at the deepest emotional level, for that is where the big life changes occur. That is where you meet yourself. Where you begin remembering who you are and who you were meant to be. I don't believe you have to be diagnosed to come to these lessons, but sometimes the catastrophic moments in life force you to focus in on the immediate.

I love Kris's book because it made me feel so many things. Familiar things. It made me laugh and reflect. And thank God, she is one of those women who has the courage and generosity to share her experience. Let's face it, life is a constant challenge. It's full of unexpected detours that no one but you can navigate. This book will be a comfort to so many who are going through the experience or who have graduated to survivor.

—**Sheryl Crow**

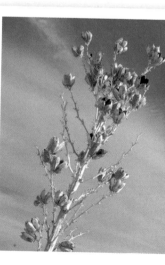

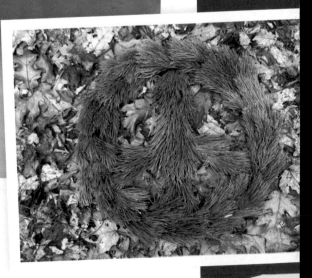

CHAPTER ONE

happy valentine's day!
you have cancer.

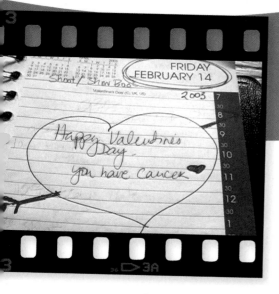

NEEDLE OFF THE RECORD.
PARTY'S OVER.
REWIND. STOP. PLAY.

February 2003. After a week of partying like a rock star at Florida's Sarasota Film Festival, where a film I was in premiered, I returned home to New York City, ready to begin a new detox and health plan. No drinking for one month—seriously. I had been burning the candle at both ends, and my body was crying out for a break. I wanted to be happier and healthier, lose a few pounds, and catch up on some much-needed sleep. Basically I was exhausted and sick and tired of complaining about it. How many times had I started a health kick only to sabotage it a few days later? It was so much easier to care for my career, business, clients, friends, family, everyone else . . . but me. This time something inside me was saying, *Enough is enough.*

So the very next day, I started my new regime by going to a yoga class. Not just any yoga but Jivamukti style—the trendy, metrospiritual workout that combines vigorous asana with chanting and kick-ass

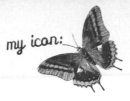
my icon:

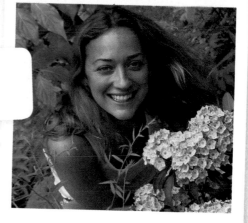

PROFILE:
KRIS CARR

AGE: Professionally, 25; legally, 30-something

HAIR COLOR: Blond

EYES: Green

HEIGHT: 5'8"

WEIGHT: 122-ish (okay, 130-plus)

HOMETOWN: Pawling, New York

OCCUPATION: Award-winning actress, photographer, and filmmaker

FAVORITE SAYING: "You want to make God laugh? Tell Her your plans!"

BEST TIP: Read this book! Highlight it, scribble in it, doodle, write down your tips, and share them with other Cancer Babes who need to giggle, sob, dance, and reflect.

music. With dreams of a cleansed and blissed-out yoga bod, I optimistically signed up for a one-month series.

In yoga you're supposed to leave your cell phone and ego at the door. On that particular day I did neither. It had been months since I'd practiced strenuous yoga, but there was a hot guy directly in front of me . . . so I acted like a professional pretzel. Hot Guy and I kept catching each other's eye, me in forearm stand, and him sneaking a peek while curled up in the child's pose. I showed off and flirted through-out the entire class—until my phone rang, which created a wave of incredulous gasps throughout the room. For those of you who have never made the mistake of shattering the Zen with your Motorola, it's totally humiliating.

The following morning I felt like a truck had hit me. It was obvious that I'd been way, way off base about my fitness level. I shrugged off the pain and went about my business, con-firming headshot appointments and booking auditions, followed by the daily slathering-on of makeup, pouring myself into tight jeans and push-up bra, and curling my blond hair into winsome locks.

I was a professional photographer and an actress. Every day I pimped the product either in front of or behind the lens. Since my recent Super Bowl victory, where I appeared in not one but two Bud Light spots, I was considered "the Julia Roberts of advertising" (accord-ing to my agent) and was temporarily in high demand. In some circles I was even considered iconic. Thousands of drunken frat boys took time out of their pepperoni pizzas and seven-layer dips to determine whether or not they'd "do" me.

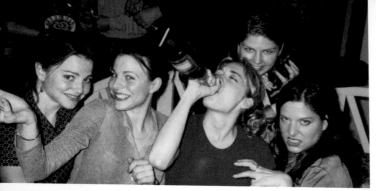

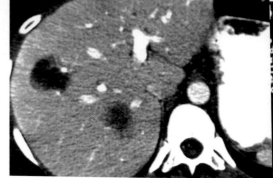

CARR, KRIS
C...
LENOX HIL

3
dB/C 4
ist Off
Opt:FSCT
tate:Surv
oCT®

The audition of the day: a commercial for a famous diet shake whose name I won't mention. It doesn't matter anyway because it turned out I was too fat for the ad and didn't get the job. How quickly my shooting star had fallen. P.S.: Think twice the next time you compare yourself to people on the boob tube or in the fashion rags. If I had a dollar for every time I've been retouched by the industrial advertising complex, I'd be living high on the hog!

Fast-forward to the evening. My muscle pain had gotten worse. Added to the mix was shortness of breath and severe abdominal cramps. Something was up. Shit! How inconvenient. My health plan had barely begun. I called my doctor the next morning.

Dr. Fabulous was like the Nobu of medicine: You couldn't get a seat unless you knew someone. Fortunately Dr. Fabulous was a big theater fan and remembered me from a buck-naked, check-out-my-birthday-suit nude scene I did in the Arthur Miller play *Mr. Peters' Connections* with Peter Falk. I saw Dr. Fabulous once or twice a year and he never failed to tell me, in a disappointed tone, how different I looked on stage; he wouldn't recognize me if he didn't know it was me. No kidding. There is a big difference between being all sexed up to play the ghost of Marilyn Monroe and looking red-nosed, bleary-eyed, and in need of serious antibiotics.

Dr. F's assistant Danielle, a real broad—

tough, feisty, and lovable—walked into the examination room and barked, "Why the hell are you here?" I told her I thought I'd fractured a rib on my first day of detox showing off for a hot guy in yoga class. She snorted and buried her hands in my abdomen. I writhed in pain. "I think it's your gallbladder," she told me. "Let's see what the doc says."

Dr. F did his usual drive-by examination and agreed that the pain was probably the result of a faulty gallbladder, which more than likely needed to be yanked, but not by him because he had vacation plans. Damn! He sent me off with a prescription for some very tasty pain drugs and ordered an ultrasound—posthaste.

Half an hour later I was lying on yet another examination table while a nameless nurse passed a scanner across my gel-covered belly. She had a mysterious half-worried, half-trying-to-look-casual expression on her face. I kept asking her what she was seeing, but she was evasive. "I am not sure. I'm having a hard time; you're very gassy." I laughed. She couldn't see my gallbladder because I was gassy? She left the room, came back with another instrument, and started scanning again. This time the seriously distressed look in her eyes made it clear that she saw something.

"What?" I asked her.

"You'll have to speak with the doctor," she said.

Something was very wrong.

DIOLOGY   C5-2 Abd/ABD**   06 Feb 03   TIs 0.4   MI 1.3   CARR, KRISTIN
1:13:17 pm   Fr #77   12.5cm   LENOX HILL RADIOLOGY
ATL   −0   Map 3
170dB/C 4
Persist Off
2D
Fr
So   −5

{ swiss cheese }

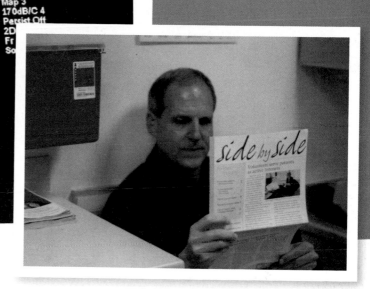

First I called my friend David to come and wait for the results with me, and then I called my dad, Ken. He quickly headed for the city. My mom stayed behind to take care of my ailing ninety-two-year-old grandmother. Finally, hours later, the doctor gave me what little news he had. The surface of my liver was covered with tumors. In fact, the pictures of my liver looked like Swiss cheese. My heart stopped. What the fuck? Next, he told me to come back in the morning for more scans and blood work. And he scheduled a next-day appointment with a gastroenterologist.

David walked me home. I sobbed the whole way. By the time we got to my apartment, my dad had arrived and was pacing the room. Dad's always been the one to go to in a mess; he's way more rational and practical than my mom, Aura. Like the time my mom caught me shoplifting. She wanted my ass hauled down to the police station to learn a lesson. Dad held my hand and brought me back to the store with the "hot" barrette and told me to apologize to the manager and tell her I'd never do it again. It was totally embarrassing and completely cured my wandering fingers. "I am really proud of you; let's get a hot chocolate," he said.

My father has always helped me come up with solutions to my problems and encouraged me to face them head-on. My mom, on the other hand, is spicy and wild-tempered (she's half Colombian). When I did something wrong, she'd lose her mind and try to melt my face with her laser-beam you-are-so-dead stare.

"What is it?" Dad asked me now. He grabbed me and shook me an inch from his face.

I burst into fresh tears. "It's my liver. They said I have tumors all over the surface of my liver."

He turned white and held me close, as if to protect me from my internal invader, as if he could squeeze the unknown disease right out of me. "Jesus Christ!" Then, "It's okay, love, we will figure this out and I will be strong for you." A rock, just like he's always been.

My father went to the bedroom to call my mom while David gave me a long hug. Ten minutes later Dad walked out red-eyed and passed me the phone. Mom was devastated. How could this be happening? That night I gave Dad my room and slept on the couch. He'd never stayed overnight at my apartment before, and since I felt guilty for possibly screwing up our lives, I wanted him to have the comfy bed.

I was fourteen years old when he adopted me. Ken Carr and my mom had been dating for five years when one sunny day he asked me the question that would change my life forever: "Would you like to call me Dad?" Though I played hard-to-get at first, secretly I was praying he'd make me his real child. My mom even bought me a special outfit for the big day: a yellow pleated skirt printed with golf balls, from Esprit. Golf is my dad's favorite sport, and though it bores me to tears, I thought the skirt would show him just how grateful I was.

Alone with my thoughts, I spent the rest of that night staring at the ceiling. My imagination ran wild. When the sun came up, I slowly got dressed. The still-constant pain of the day before had numbed my entire being, but I didn't care; my mind was focused on the slew of tests that lay ahead.

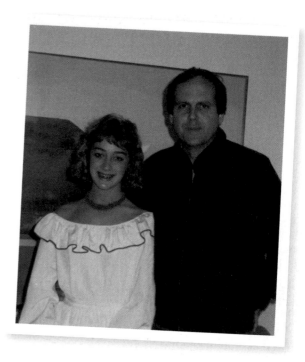

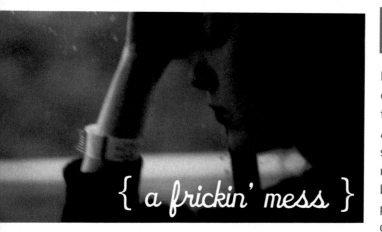

{ a frickin' mess }

Dr. Semi-Fabulous was placed in charge of my case because Dr. Fabulous was doing whatever doctors do on vacation. Dr. S's singsongy, noncommittal tone made me feel terminal. I searched his face for some kind of clue but got nothing. He threw out a few possi-

bilities: focal nodular hyperplasia, multiple adenomas. "We just don't know." A needle biopsy through my rib cage would determine for sure. As it turned out, Dr. S and my dad went to the same college, Syracuse University (go Orangemen). After what seemed like hours of the banal small talk and topical chitchat that guys pursue when they're avoiding the real issue, my dad asked to talk to the doctor alone. Oh God! I excused myself and headed to the bathroom, along the way running into feisty physician's assistant Danielle. We hugged, and she asked how I was. She had the same look in her eyes that the sonogram nurse had given me.

"What do you think it is? Seriously, what

is your hunch?" I asked, even though I wasn't ready to hear what my deep dark thoughts feared, and she knew it. So she positioned her answer as a question. "What do you think of when you think of tumors, many, many tumors?"

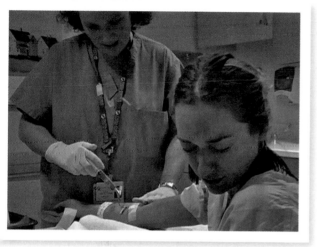

"The C-word," I replied.

"Yup."

Panic. The room started to spin. What was going on inside my body? Cancer is such a frightening word. I imagined myself hairless and clinging to life. How could this be happening to me? Cancer happened to other people. People you read about, not people you knew and loved, certainly not yourself. I was only thirty-one, young and vibrant. I was a Bud Girl, for Christ's sake! I felt like I was staring down the barrel of a gun, waiting to find out how many bullets were inside.

Over the next several days, I was in and out of the hospital for a battery of tests, including the aforementioned biopsy. There was no way I was going to sit alone in my apartment waiting for the results; I'd have snapped. So I grabbed Crystal, my cat, and spent the night at my parents' house in Connecticut. At 5:45 a.m. we woke up to a blizzard, but my dad shuffled

us all into the car anyway. My appointment wasn't until 9:00 a.m. but, by Dad's calculations, "New York's gonna be a frickin' mess." As always, he was right. We piled into the Expedition and headed to the city.

My whole body needed to be scanned, including my brain. Great. It didn't take me long to become an expert at CAT scans, MRIs, and radiology. I figured out in short order exactly which locker to use for my clothes, which direction the gown needed to face, and how to tie it and keep my dignity. On that particular snowy day, Nurse Mildred—DRED being the operative syllable—escorted me to the machine. MilDRED hated me. I stood for every dissatisfaction and frustration in her life. MilDRED was bored and depressed, and she didn't try to hide the fact that she hated every minute of working in a cancer hospital.

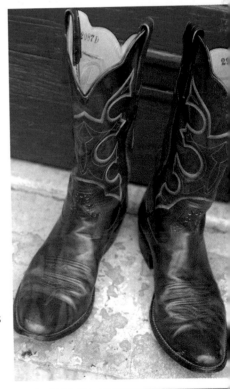

MilDRED walked five paces in front of me. I trailed behind dressed in my gown and chocolate-brown cowboy boots. She was not pleased.

"Do you want hospital slippers?" she deadpanned.

"The boots are fine," I replied.

I wore my cowboy boots every day and I certainly wasn't going to abandon them in my hour of need. They represented my fantasy life, a life of freedom on the range with a porch swing and a handsome, yet handy, cowboy at my side. I was not going to let MilDRED take the boots or the dream away from me.

{ the tunnel }

When encased in a fluorescent MRI coffin for two hours, the mind has a tendency to wander into the darkest crevices of the imagination. I began to ponder the human brain and remembered being told in biology class that we consciously use only 10 percent of its power. If that's true, how is the rest used? Is there a portion of the brain that sends

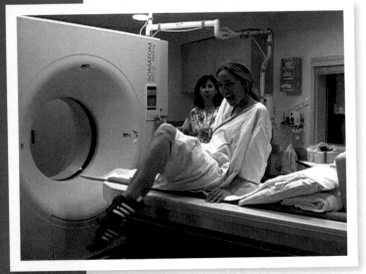

messages throughout the body to heal it? Isn't it miraculous that when you break a bone, your body knows how to fuse it back together? Is it possible to slip a message in there somehow? I felt like I was on to something.

There must be a way to code a message that I could sew into the fabric of my brain. Reverse the tumors. Reverse the tumors. I began to meditate on the command. I was visualizing, praying, pleading. Why hadn't I worked on a better relationship with God, Goddess, or whoever the heck is up there? Was it too late? I felt kinda guilty and spanked for the shallow-

ness of my usual requests: that acting job that I'd just die if I didn't get, or the destruction of the all-too-accurate scale at the gym. Now I was praying for my life and the powers that be were laughing. Ha-ha.

Just then the tray I was resting on began to move me toward the light. I never imagined it would be this way at the end, with MilDRED waiting for me on the other side.

After the tunnel trip I met up with my mom, dad, and younger sister, Leslie, all sitting in the hospital's waiting room. The room was full of people, much older than me, male and female, with and without family, all awaiting the arrival of Dr. Guru Specialist. Every door that opened, every lab coat that glided by held the promise of the Guru. I took a seat next to Leslie and started punching my boot, nervous as a cat. Was I breathing? Was my heart beating? Yes, I could feel it throbbing, racing, and throwing itself against my rib cage. Finally the sea parted and the Guru appeared. I immediately tried to read his expression. Was it good, bad, what? Was he smiling? How fast was he walking? Did he pause at the chair before sitting? *Was I going to die?* He paused! Shit!

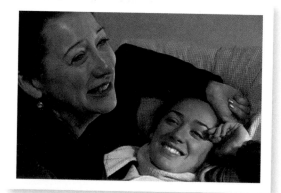

Mom and Me

{dead woman walking}

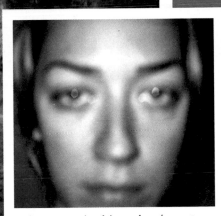

self portrait taken 1 hour after diagnosis

The doctor started his explanation with the word *Well*—a loaded word if ever there was one. It is most frequently used in such situations as breakups, layoffs, and bad medical news. Fasten your seat belt when the head of the transplant unit at Mount Sinai begins his sentence with the word *Well*. "Well, we didn't find them in your bones or spleen, but there seem to be about ten more tumors in both lungs." Silence. A wave of nausea flooded my body. My recent emotional narcolepsy promoted itself to emotional paralysis.

I excused myself to the restroom, and as I rose from my chair three words came to my mind: *Dead Woman Walking*. I locked myself in the bathroom and stared in the mirror in shock, fighting, fighting, fighting back the tears. How would I pull it together and get back out there? Cold water. I began to fill the sink with cold water. I soaked my hands in it, then my face, and as I submerged a gentle voice from down in my gut said, *No*. As family lore has it, my first spoken word was not *Mommy* or *Daddy*, but *No*. I took a deep breath and went back out for a second helping of horror.

My clan was intensely huddled around Guru. And the verdict was . . . epithelioid hemangio-endothelioma. Translation: *Holy shit!* Try to say that three times fast. You can't, so let's call it EHE for short. It's an extremely rare vascular cancer affecting the lining of the blood vessels in my liver and lungs. Stage IV. Nationwide, there are approximately two to three hundred cases of EHE diagnosed annually. It typically appears in multiple sites, and nobody knows how it happens. Great! Pass the chardonnay.

Next topic: liver transplant. Not only had a train hit me, but now it was speeding away, dragging me behind. Because tumors had also been found in another area of my body, I was not a high priority on the donor list—why waste a liver on me when the cancer had already spread to both lungs? Just as well. I wanted to keep all my bits and pieces anyway, thank you very much. I plan on leaving with what I came with. My dad, ever the optimist, quickly asked if anyone in the family could donate half a liver, if a match existed. There has been much success with partial transplants, and my clan was eager to help. Nope. In my case the tumors would probably pollute the new half, and we'd be back to square one.

The "C" word, me . . . how is that possible? I'm young, healthy, and active. I was good, I followed the rules, ate right, exercised, drank in moderation, I say please and thank you and leave 20%, I'm vegetarian for moral reasons, for God's sake, I'm a Democrat! I did all the right things.

Why me? How does this happen?

Next, my mother began a line of questioning, and I could just smell the direction it was taking.

"How old a liver can you use?" she asked.

"There have been positive results in livers up to ninety-two years old," the Guru responded.

"Oh," my mother replied. "How long can it be on ice for?" She was offering my grandma's liver! My grandma: at the time still very much alive, and still very much a pain in my mother's ass.

"Mom! She isn't even dead yet!" I pictured Mom brandishing a pillow next to Granny's bed, a cooler by her side, and burst into laughter. Guru was not amused. In fact, if I had been him, I would have alerted the authorities.

Since I was asymptomatic, the Guru recommended a "watch and wait, let the tumors declare their intentions before attacking the shit out of them," approach, at least for the next two months. He wanted to gauge how the cancer was moving: steady, slow, or fast. Why couldn't I have a popular cancer? No, I had to get a rare cancer that only affects about 0.1 percent of the population. There would be no groups for me, no walks, no ribbons, no sisterhood bullshit, nothing. In fact, although studies are under way, there is no cure and no definitive treatment for EHE. What! Why? I guess the answer to that is pretty obvious. Why spend time and valuable money on a disease that affects only a few people? I used to celebrate my uniqueness; now it seemed like a total detriment to my survival.

Patience has never been one of my strengths. The idea of casually sitting on a time bomb was about as appealing to me as sliding down a razor blade into a cold pool of alcohol. And yet a part of me was relieved and grateful that my disease could be slow moving. I mean, the one thing that all cancer patients pray for is time, and for the moment it looked like I had it. Plus, I had no desire to start some crazy experimental treatment right away. Becoming an observational lab rat was definitely not my cup of tea.

As I fought back tears, I asked if there was anything I could do. "No, just try and live a normal life," Dr. Guru said. Earth to Dr. Guru, come in, Dr. Guru. Was he high? How the hell could I do that? How could I live with cancer without thinking of dying every day? It was just so weird. I didn't look sick, I didn't feel sick, and yet there was so much cancer in me. "If you want to, focus on building your immune system through diet and lifestyle," he added.

I quickly perked up. He'd just thrown me a crumb of control. I could do that! I could participate! I could educate myself and help my body out! Shit, maybe I could figure out how to get rid of this thing on my own (I've always had a rather inflated sense of myself).

Dr. Guru didn't know it, but in that moment he planted the seeds for a personal revolution.

Right then and there, I vowed to take that crumb and turn it into a cake. I was not gonna kick back and wait for the unknown. I was going to dive in and become a full-time healing junkie!

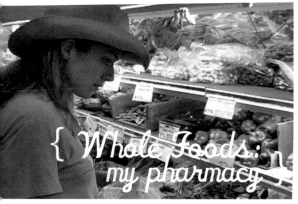

{ *Whole Foods: my pharmacy* }

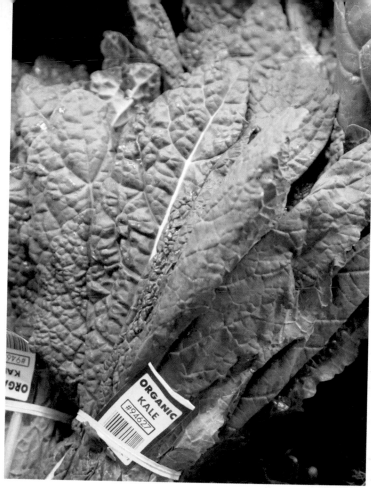

Next stop: Whole Foods, the organic grocery superstore. The four of us piled back into my dad's Expedition and sped down Seventh Avenue. My family was in shock. Though slightly empowered, I was still extremely numb. As I rolled down the window and the blast of winter air slapped my face, tears began to flow down my cheeks like water from an overflowing tub, calmly and consistently. My facial expression never changed.

My mother raced around the store frantically filling two shopping carts with every organic piece of produce she could get her hands on. If it was leafy and green, it went into our cart. My mind was so overloaded, I couldn't even muster a protest at the sight of the dinosaur kale in my mom's desperate little hands. What would we even do with this scary-looking vegetable? If the cancer didn't kill me, this plant certainly would. My sister and I grabbed books, vitamins, herbal potions, and candles (I had to relax, right? Stress is bad! RELAX!). I'll admit I did throw in a few items that had nothing to do with cancer but I was too cheap to buy for myself. My parents would have written a check for forever to make it all go away; they certainly wouldn't protest over a tube of $30 Dr. Hauschka face cream.

Though I was showing up late for Cancer College, at least I was enrolled—and determined to ace all my tests!

That night I went to bed feeling more alone than I'd ever felt in my life. The next day

I woke up and started work on my survival plan. The first appointment I scheduled after they put a name to the face of my cancer was a second opinion, followed by a third and a fourth. I met some of the best cancer doctors in the country. Though each one had a different theory and different approach, they all agreed that in my case "watch and wait" was the way to go. If you wanted a cancer treatment that would really make you frustrated, this was it.

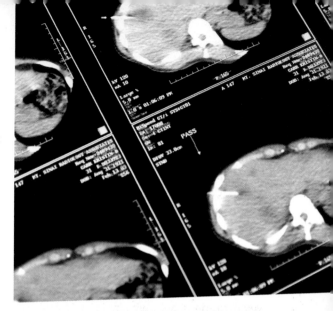

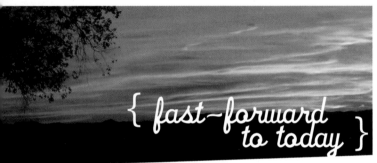

{ *fast-forward to today* }

So much has changed since February 14, 2003. I pulled a Dumpster up to my life and totally renovated my way of being. I still have cancer. The doctors use the term *indolent* when describing the tumors now. Definition: "Lethargic; not showing any interest or making any effort" (sounds like me at fifteen). Whether I like it or not, they're a part of me. But I am happy to say that (for the time being) the cancer is stable—that is, not growing. It's like a light switch that's turned off, and there is a good chance it'll stay that way. Cancer as a chronic disease? Chronic diseases are herpes and diabetes, not the big C. It was just so hard to understand. Like most people (doctors included), I was still caught up in the militaristic shock-and-awe, win-the-war approach.

But cancer has changed, and so have I. Life goes on, even becomes normal again. I refused to let cancer wreck my party. There are just too many cool things to do and plan and live for.

I hate using the G-word—you know, cancer is a "Gift." Yuck. It isn't! There is no return receipt, and it certainly isn't a present I'd give to you. "Happy holidays! Ooh, just what I wanted, *cancer*, you really shouldn't have." Cancer isn't a puppy, a pony, a new doll, or a shiny truck. Cancer isn't something to say thank you for, but it can be a catalyst. I finally had permission to take risks, put myself first, and dump my baggage. Yes, it may have been Louis Vuitton, but it still had to go! Why had I neglected myself for so long? I had an inner voice that knew better, so why had I ignored it?

It's all a process. And change takes time. Some days I really understand the need for kindness and self-compassion. Other days I frantically try to push against the river, or I just break down and sob. If yoga (now a more mature practice, no flirting or disrupting) teaches me anything, it's to be flexible. Cancer is a strong wind that can completely uproot you if you don't sway with it.

Cancer made me say, "Screw it and do it" (annoyingly clichéd but true)—I mean, what was I waiting for? Out with the old world order, in with the new. I made some pretty radical changes (which I'll tell you about throughout this book). In a nutshell, I quit my job, moved, got really healthy, met a wonderful man, and guess what? Cancer or not, I got hitched!

I also took a huge artistic leap. When I was first diagnosed, there wasn't much in the way of books or movies that dealt with the situations and problems facing young women with cancer. Everything was geared toward either kids or people much older than me, and most of it was either really sappy or really depressing. I hadn't raised children, gotten to the end of my career, entered into a second marriage, or buried my parents yet. I was just getting started!

This is crap. I decided cancer needed a makeover, and I was just the gal to do it! So as a creative outlet, I began writing and filming my journey. I documented everything and everyone—the physicians, teachers, gurus, alternative doctors, and alternative quacks. The camera was my buddy. I talked, it listened, no judgment. The lens allowed me to vent and say the scary things I didn't want to admit to anyone. At times it provided distance from my drama by allowing me to be an artist instead of a patient.

After a while I longed to hear inspirational stories from other women. The only problem was that I hated the idea of support groups (great for some, not for me). I pictured them like some awkward teary cancer AA. "Hi, my name is Kris and I have cancer," followed by, in unison, "Hi, Kris!" No thanks. In truth, I was too chicken for that kind of thing. Yes, I needed support, but it had to be on my terms. When you're healthy, you think cancer is so far away. But when you get sick, you realize that it's all around; you just have to open your eyes. So I picked up the phone and called everyone in my Elvis Presley (a souvenir from Graceland) address book. "Do you know any young women with cancer?" The e-mails and phone numbers began to pour in, and my first Cancer Babe playdates were scheduled!

{ cancer babes }

Cancer connected me to women I would never have met otherwise: women who understood me in a way that no one else could. Some of them even let me film their stories for my documentary, which I named *Crazy Sexy Cancer*. The name concerned some people at first. Was I being flip, disrespectful, inappropriate? No. I still had a sense of humor, which I wasn't going to amputate just because there suddenly was this really serious thing in my life. I didn't want to lose myself. I was still crazy, sexy (sometimes), curious, silly, and struggling. Poking fun at cancer helped me cope with it.

At last, I felt normal again! Normal and successful: Apparently The Learning Channel also wondered where the stories of young women with cancer were hiding. So in the fall of 2006 (a month after I got married) they bought my film. In 2007 *Crazy Sexy Cancer* had its world premiere at the South by Southwest Film Festival in Austin, Texas. It was a hit! Who knew cancer could be such a big box-office draw?

The idea for this book came shortly thereafter. *Crazy Sexy Cancer Tips* is more than just a memoir; it's a collection of facts, hints, hell-yeahs, how-tos, and know-hows for all you glorious Cancer Babes out there.

These are fundamental, practical, silly, real, fun, crazy, sexy ways to live your life—with cancer. Because it can be done. You can do it. Now smile, lady, you're not alone.

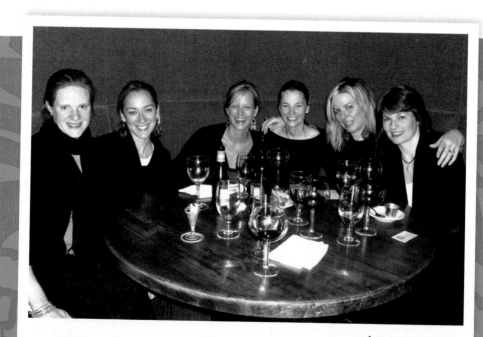

A posse powwow

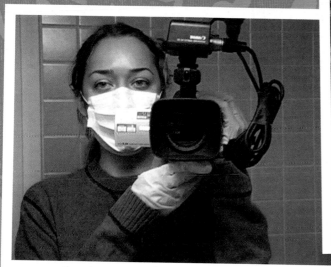

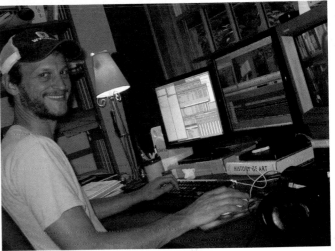

CRAZY SEXY CANCER — A REVIEW

Kris Carr has created a brilliant, gorgeous and staggering documentary about her journey through cancer. Determined to prove that her life is not over just because the type of cancer she has is "incurable," she is willing to try anything. A newly minted "healing junkie," she delves into the world of New Age health seminars and alternative therapies. Her still healthy sense of humor thumbs its nose at the idea that she will never be cured.

Carr responds by creating a network of cancer chicks to foster a no-bullshit attitude to deal with the largely stigmatized disease. Befriending hip cancer heroes Jackie "Fuck Cancer" Farry and the Zammett sisters helps her to balance the loneliness of having such a rare condition. These women show cancer who's boss, sometimes through the power of sheer orneriness. *Crazy Sexy Cancer* is essentially a crash course in "Welcome to Having Cancer, Population: You."

--Tammy Lynn Bolton

CREATE A
cancer posse

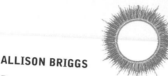

ALLISON BRIGGS

Breast cancer survivor. Founder of The Rack Pack, an organization that assists young women diagnosed with cancer.

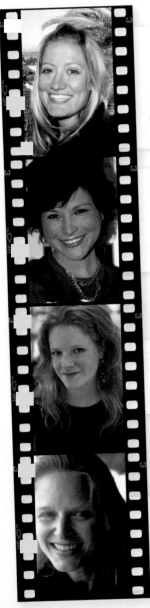

DIEM BROWN

Star of *MTV's Real World/ Road Rules Challenge* and founder of Live for the Challenge.

ERIN ZAMMETT RUDDY

Author, columnist, and cancer activist.

HEIDI ADAMS

Founder of Planet Cancer, a community of young adults with cancer.

Create your own sassy support group/cancer stitch-and-bitch. My posse makes me howl! Our conversations range from everyday stuff like dieting, boyfriends, jobs, and plans for the future to funny cancer escapades and deep "what-ifs" that only a CB (Cancer Babe) can understand. My crew teaches me that it's okay to still have normal problems and dramas. 'Cause underneath it all we're still girls.

Create your own posse as soon as possible, and keep adding to it as time goes on. There is a lot of crap you have to cope with, and your posse can help. Plus, you'll find yourself trading valuable tricks of the trade.

Ask your doctor if he or she can connect you with other young women your age. Start networking with everyone you can think of. Once you start asking and searching, you will find other women, sometimes right in your own neighborhood. Some of mine contributed a lot of their stories and tips for this book. Check out who they are, 'cause I'll be singing their praises throughout the book. Notice that each one has a graphic identifier—whenever you see one of these icons next to a tip, you'll know who it came from. Thanks, Posse!

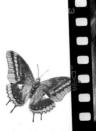

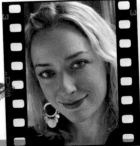

JACKIE FARRY

Rock-and-roll tour manager, Fuck Cancer organizer.

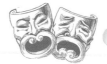

ONI FAIDA LAMPLEY

Playwright, actress.

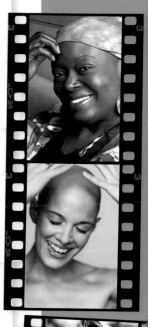

JODI SAX

Founder of LifeLab, a New York City support community for young adult cancer survivors in their twenties and thirties.

SHARON BLYNN

Model, cancer activist, founder of Bald Is Beautiful.

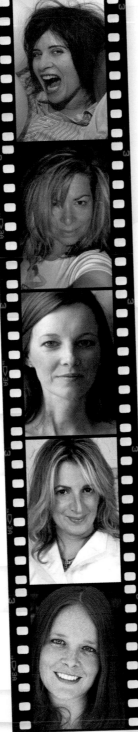

LINDSAY BECK

Young mom and founder of Fertile Hope, a fertility resource for women with cancer.

SUZANNE DONALDSON

Photo director at *Glamour* magazine, my beautiful cousin.

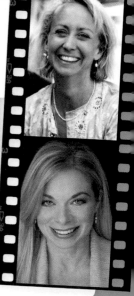

MARISA ACOCELLA MARCHETTO

Celebrated cartoonist and author of *Cancer Vixen*.

CancerVixen

TERRI COLE

Licensed psychotherapist; television acting teacher at New York University; talk-show host.

MELISSA GONZALEZ

Erin Zammett Ruddy's sister, young mom, cancer survivor.

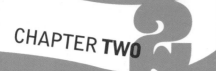

CHAPTER TWO

holy shit! I HAVE CANCER.
NOW WHAT?

{ *breathe* }

Okay, so the shit just hit the fan. Take a deep breath, get grounded, and center yourself. Like Alice in Cancerland, you're falling down a dark and creepy rabbit hole. Doctors are spewing lots of information, most of which probably goes in one ear and out the other. Why? Because when you're newly diagnosed with cancer, this is what you hear: "Blah, blah, CANCER, blah, blah, YOU ARE GOING TO DIE, blah, blah CANCER."

So here it is. Yesterday you were a normal civilian; today you are a cancer patient survivor. Getting diagnosed throws your entire universe into a free fall. There's no sugarcoating it: Cancer is a devastating blow, one that takes time to process. My shrink taught me that

cancer patients go through the same post-traumatic stress disorder as soldiers or rape victims.

At first I thought she was being awfully dramatic (though I appreciated

20

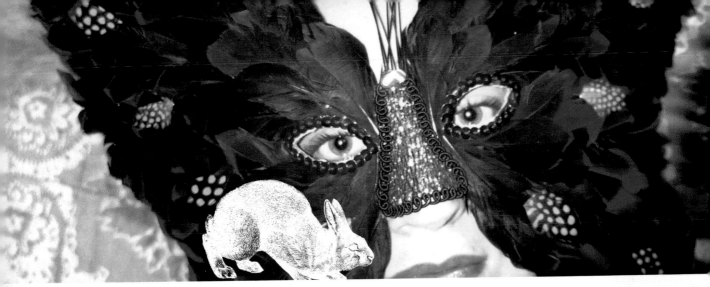

it), but then it made sense. I was in total shock after my diagnosis. To be honest, that shock lasted several years, and even though I never had treatment and manage the cancer on my own, at times I am still overcome by it.

A quick look at the online public encyclopedia Wikipedia puts the idea into an even broader perspective: "PTSD is normally associated with trauma such as violent crimes, rape, and war experience. However, there have been a growing number of reports of PTSD among cancer survivors and their relatives (Smith 1999, Kangas 2002). Cancer as trauma is multifaceted, includes multiple events that can cause distress, and like combat, is often characterized by extended duration with a potential for recurrence and a varying immediacy of life-threat (Smith 1999)." On top of that you can also suffer from PTSD after being attacked by a vicious dog, shark, or mountain lion. That's it—no more waterskiing near the Great Barrier Reef or hikes in Patagonia for me.

All of us who have heard the three deafening words *you have cancer* struggle to figure out how and why it happened. What did I do

wrong? We desperately want answers. Sometimes we may even want to blame someone or something for crashing us into our own mortality and forcing us to face it. It's crazy-making!

So I'm not saying it's easy, but now is not the time to lose your mind and curl up in a ball or go postal. You need your wits about you, sister. There are lots of decisions to make, and the more grounded you are, the more sensible your choices will be. If I'd listened to one of the first doctors I talked to, I'd have ended up sliced, fried, and hauling around not one but three organs that didn't belong to me! Needless to say, I don't think I'd be here, writing this book, and sharing my story with you.

There are no hard-and-fast rules on how to deal with a diagnosis. I wish I could give you a road map, but I can't. No two cancers are the same, and neither are the experiences that surround them. Remember, when you're newly diagnosed, everyone who loves you is freaked out, not just you. Friendships shift. Family roles and dynamics change, sometimes forever.

So what *do* you do? Everything you can to create joy in your world. Just because you have cancer doesn't mean you can't go out, enjoy life, and be you. Unless you're in treatment and feel like a truck has hit you, in which case you are a queen and for the time being you get the biggest piece of emotional birthday cake. But whether you're feeling fine or not, never think of yourself as a Sick Person. So often we wait for all our ducks to be in a row, our closets to be neat and tidy, and our endless to-do lists to be checked off before we allow ourselves to have fun. We believe that only after we get all our "stuff" done can we take a deep breath and live.

Well, cancer doesn't wait for order. In fact, it thrives on chaos. Breathe now. Burn the lists, and let the dust bunnies roll like tumbleweeds. Narrow your focus to what really matters: you. Cancer is unknown territory. Will life ever be the same? I hate to burst your bubble, but no. Can you still drink wine? Maybe. Dance on tables? Yes. Go on vacation? Absolutely. Be "normal"? Why would you want to be that?

tip no.2

FIND AND VISIT
a personal refuge

Where and what makes you happy?
Figure it out and spend some time in that space. If you don't know someplace that makes you happy, then this is a good time for some soul searching. Is there a spot in your house or neighborhood, a beach walk, a park, a beautiful drive, a particular view or vista that always relaxes you? Wherever or whatever it is—go there. For me it's the woods.

When I needed a vacation from my thoughts, I would buy a bus ticket and head upstate to "hippieville" (better known as Woodstock, New York) for long mountain hikes and a chance to breathe in the crisp air and walk until all the fear was out. Then I'd head back home. Sometimes I'd get a room in the bed-and-breakfast in town and stay overnight. When I strolled around looking for a place to have dinner, I'd pretend that I was someone else. Since nobody knew me, I could pretend to be healthy; I could make up a new story and give myself a break from the real one. Maybe it was denial, but it helped. Even if it's just for a few hours, find a way to take a mental hiatus from cancer.

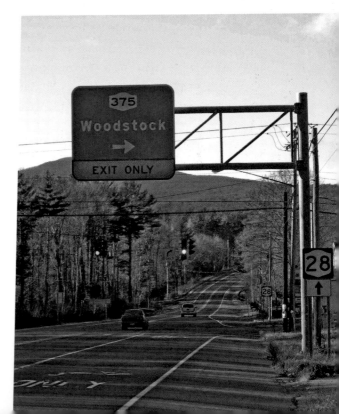

tip no.3

CREATE A
sacred space

It may sound like total tree-hugging hippie new-age crystal crap, but it helps to have a corner of your home that feels sacred. It can be as simple as a candle on your nightstand or some fresh flowers on your kitchen table.

For me a breakfast-in-bed table (which had never been used for its intended purpose) made a perfect little altar. I covered it with pictures of my favorite people, candles, incense, my grandma's rosary, some seashells from a beach I wanted to see again, and a rock from my mom's garden. I placed it in a corner of my apartment where two red walls came together (for dramatic effect) and plopped a groovy satin pillow in front of it.

For the first year after my diagnosis, I would spend about ten minutes every day just being there: feeling my butt on the pillow, taking deep breaths, and talking to myself. Pep talks, prayers, confessions—to a fly on the wall, I probably looked like some senile whack job. But I was learning who I was, meeting my inner voice. In the beginning it was a soft little whimper; now it's a thunderous roar.

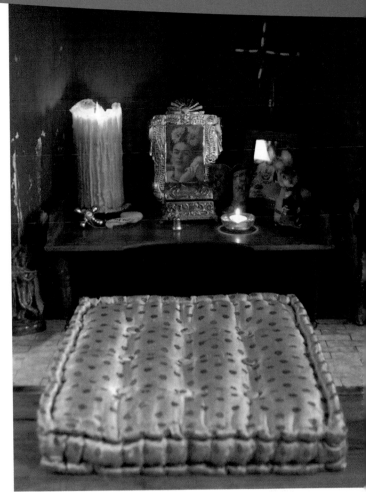

tip no.4

REMOVE THESE WORDS
FROM YOUR DAILY SPEECH:

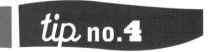

maybe   sure
i don't know
and—this is the best one—
you decide

Before cancer I was kinda voiceless about a lot of important things in my life. My common response to questions or decisions was, "Whatever you want is fine with me." Now I can get pretty mouthy 'cause I'm no longer afraid to say what I want and ask for what I need. And guess what? It's okay to put yourself first. Everyone else takes care of number one, so why can't you? It's not selfish! Cancer isn't killing me, it's just forcing me to grow up.

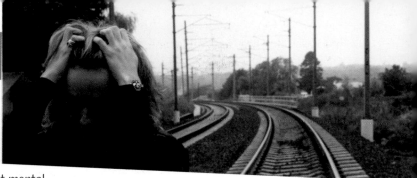

TAKE TIME TO
mourn

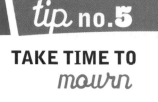

Living with cancer is all about mental management. The creepy thoughts will always try to slide under the radar. You'll be slicing the Thanksgiving turkey and thinking about how to word your gravestone, watching TV but imagining who your husband or partner will hook up with after you're gone (you may even get mad during this little fantasy, especially if you imagine him with someone younger and prettier than you!). The first few years of my diagnosis I swear I had an alternate thought track playing on a loop in my mind. Thank God no one ever asked me what I was thinking about! How I wished I could go back to the carefree innocence that I had taken for granted before the cancer talon popped my little bubble.

Unfortunately there will always be a B.C. (Before Cancer Hijacked My Life), and sadly we can never go back.

Give yourself time to process the diagnosis and let it sink in.

It will feel like a death at first, a loss of freedom and safety. But cancer won't always be your first and last thought of the day. I promise. Life moves on. Taxes still need to be paid, your laundry still needs to be washed, and the oil in your car still has to be changed every three thousand miles. As life returns to normal, you may come to the acceptance that, like it or not, cancer is just another thing in your life you have to roll with. It might even become another interesting piece of your puzzle that separates you in a good way. Once you go head-to-head with cancer, there is nothing you can't do!

tip no.6

EXPECT THE "WHY ME?"
cancer blues

My struggle to understand Why me? has led me down many roads. Understanding the complexities of cancer is a full-time job, and none of us applies for the position! You may—no, you will—get the Why me? cancer blues, and that's normal and totally expected. Talk it through with someone you trust. Find the strongest shoulder and cry on it.

Get mad, sad, desperate, numb, whatever, just go there and don't bottle it up.

However, be careful not to spiral. Set a limit. If you find yourself in the same pajamas from sunrise to sunset and back to sunrise, surrounded by take-out cartons and movies like *Beaches* or *Wit*—it's okay, give yourself a break, and then snap out of it! Your mourning just became wallowing, and wallowing gets you nowhere. Here's a trick: Make a three-day rule. Allow me to elaborate.

the **3-DAY** rule

Have you ever heard the saying about fish and houseguests? After three days they both start to stink. Well, so does wallowing. I know this sounds harsh, but it's true. Try to explore and indulge the feelings for no more than three days, and then move on. Not to say you can't visit those emotions again. Cancer is a roller

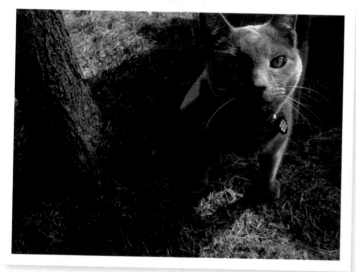

coaster: One minute you're up, the next you're plummeting to the ground.

Your mental state really helps your physical condition, so give yourself the Three-Day Rule and get back in the saddle.

'Cause, lady, you are a survivor and someone who goes the distance; this isn't about the sprint—it's about the long haul.

Every day we decide how to use our time and energy. Use it wisely. Listen to your inner mother. She knows what's best for you. She knows when you need more sleep, a good nurturing meal, a hug; she knows who you should be hanging out with and who wastes your time. She even knows when you need a good old-fashioned time-out. Don't be rebellious; listen.

Example: Early in my diagnosis my mom came for a cheer-up visit. The curtains were drawn and the take-out cartons were jockeying for the closest position to the remote. Intervention time! Mom quickly hosed me off and jammed my cat Crystal and me in the car for a weekend of TLC in Connecticut. It was a hot summer day, and we were soon stuck in bumper-to-bumper traffic. My sweet little usually mellow kitty was having a total shit fit, screaming her head off. Finally I snapped. Before I could even stop myself, I grabbed her carrier and let out a shrill that should have shattered the car windows. Now, mind you, I am a vegan and an animal lover, but in a moment of rage mixed with exhaustion and cancer fear I began to shake the cage with the desperation of a claustrophobic prisoner behind bars.

My mother didn't say a word. She just waited for me to calm down and get back into my seat. The pressure of it all just collapsed in on me: no laughter, love, or rational-speak could have made it better. What I really wanted to say (scream) was, I have cancer, this is so unfair and I'm really scared! Nevertheless, I felt like I was starting to purge the woe-is-me devil. (P.S.: My cat is fine; she just gave me a dirty look, waited about five minutes, and then started howling again.)

The next day I still felt like emotional shit, but I forced myself to go for a run. As I sweated it out, the nasty despair started to lift. That's when I established the Three-Day Rule.

Dealing with the depression was far more painful than the actual cancer. I'll admit I've been pretty lucky: "Cancer light," I call it. This silly disease doesn't stop me from living a normal life. Yes, that might change one day, but if I wasted my time focusing on that possibility now I'd just be missing all the fun stuff.

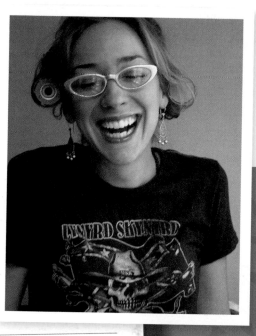

JOURNAL ENTRY

I thought I was safe. I thought I had a grace period to explore the borders of my youth. I used to pride myself on walking the edge, dangling, and recovering right before the big drop. I got high on it. But cancer gets the last laugh. Funny, I always knew something big would happen in my life, I just didn't know it would be like this! Follow your gut. How do I find stability in the midst of un-safety? How do I make balance in my world?

How is it going to be okay when everything is so not okay?

Excuse me, waitress, I want to order again. I want to go back to a time where math and logic made sense of it all. I can't believe I'm going to say this, but I want rules and curfews, phone time from 9-10 only after I finish my homework.

I want protection.

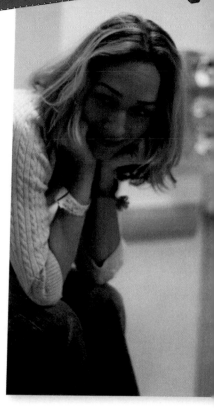

tip no. 7

GET A *shrink!*

There are oceans of feelings that you need to process as a result of your diagnosis. Therapists, support groups, and Cancer Posses (like my glam pack) can help you cope. Surrounding yourself with family and friends can be a great source of strength—but be mindful of their needs, too. They may only be able to comfort you in moderation. Remember, they have their own stuff to deal with; don't expect them to be sitting by the phone for your 24/7 Holy Shit Hotline.

Some of your feelings may seem totally irrational, but underneath the ridiculous there always lies an important jewel. I went through a phase where I was riddled with jealousy and resentment of so-called healthy people. I was an irrational wreck! Mad is much easier for me to express than sad, and rage felt damn good, so I judged everybody walking down the street. All pedestrians were carefree, flower-smelling lucky idiots; I was the sick one. I felt isolated; no longer could I play in their cancer-free sandbox. Instead I was alone on the seesaw, with no pal to push me up when I was feeling so down.

the **THERAPY** *couch*

I knew it was time to plant my ass on the therapy couch when random strangers inspired violent fantasies. I wanted to trip the beautiful (and skinny) brunette with the ice cream cone and blasé attitude. Doesn't she know that she is one lick away from cancer! I wanted to trip her and kick her and make her cry. The funny thing was, I didn't wish that she had it instead of me; I wished she had it, too. I wanted there to be some kind of consistency in the world, a universal through-line. She ate it or drank it or lived by the same toxic dump or her genetic code was scrambled, too. Whatever the cause, we'd be sick together.

But life is messy and inconsistent (which is ultimately why it's so fabulous). Yet for a Virgo who hates change (August 31 is my birthday, feel free to send a card), it can also be very unsettling! I knew that I needed to talk about my misplaced anger (shrink term) or I'd end up in a women's correctional facility. So once again I picked up the phone and networked. I had no idea how many of my friends were in therapy! This made me feel like I wasn't the only nutter out there. I cried through my shrink's entire box of Kleenex-brand tissues (with lotion) at the first session. But seventy-five clams later I felt better. A deadweight (no pun intended) had been lifted off my chest. "See you next week!"

27

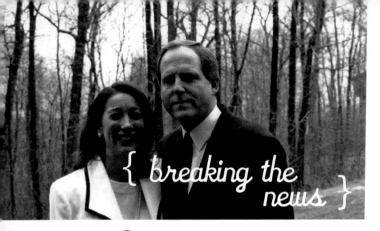

{ breaking the news }

For me, breaking the news and talking about cancer was like listening to the sound of fake nails dragging across a chalkboard. Excruciating. No matter how much I practiced or rehearsed (I have cancer, I have cancer, I have cancer), it was a total disaster! Unfortunately there's no easy way to do it. So let's learn from my mistakes and start with what not to do first, shall we?

After the doctors found that the tumors had spread to my lungs, my family and I needed to regroup big-time. Though we were fairly sure I had cancer, we held out hope that there was a mistake, that the doctors had accidentally read someone else's scans or that these strange little lesions were surprisingly benign. Denial was to act as our life preserver until the results of my biopsy were read.

I felt like a scared kid who just wanted to hide under her parents' bed. I wanted to be protected by the grown-ups, to be fed grilled-cheese sandwiches and tomato soup with goldfish crackers, to be told that if I finished my lunch it would all go away.

My parents wanted me close, too, which wasn't going to be hard since I temporarily moved back in with them and had Velcroed myself and Crystal to my old high school bed. They did everything for me, and I didn't make one move without them. The only time I was alone was after they tucked me in at night (yes, they actually tucked me in. At thirty-one I had totally regressed).

February 14, Valentine's Day. The phone rang, I answered it; the results were in. There were no mistakes, no possible this or that or Let's just make sure. There was only cancer and a lot of it. My mom was sitting by my side on the sofa, crossing all fingers and toes, asking for angels and praying to the gods of all the religions just in case the one we believed in was a chump.

In the next breath I leveled her. "IT'S END STAGE. I NEED A LAWYER. YOU CAN HAVE MY JEWELRY!" Do not give your loved ones

A SLIGHT TICKLE

A note about biopsies: The nurse who performed the procedure promised me that it would just slightly tickle. OH, REALLY? Since when does a ten-foot-long needle shoved through your rib cage and into your liver tickle? Tip: Take what the doctors and nurses say about pain and double it. Unless they've been through it, they really don't know.

a heart attack by delivering news this way. My poor mother was obliterated.

Each family member was harder to break the news to than the last, but nothing was as hard as telling my grandmother. As I mentioned earlier, she was at the end of her life, and she knew it. My mom didn't want her to die in a nursing home or a cold hospital room, so she took her in. Can you imagine facing the reality of losing your mother and possibly your daughter at the same time? My mother's inner strength was and still is staggering.

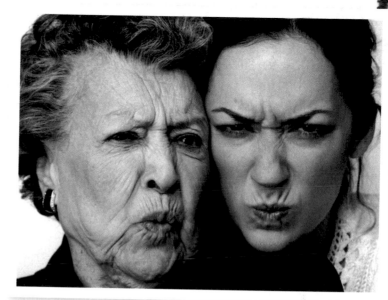

Back to my grandma. How could I talk about death with one of the people I cherished the most, especially since, for her, it was right around the corner? My mom shared with me that Grandma knew her time was coming and was actually okay with dying. She imagined what the world behind the sun looked like, and apparently it wasn't so bad. When I heard this, a boulder-size lump closed my throat and hot tears boiled in my eyes. I wasn't ready for my grandma to die, and I also wasn't ready to tell her that I might be right behind her.

CANCER ARMOR

Ladies, this advice may sound fluffy, but it's so helpful . . . before you tell the important people in your life, look your best. Get an eyebrow wax, a manicure, and a new outfit. I call it Cancer Armor. People you tell are going to discreetly and not-so-discreetly try to see the cancer, so dazzle them instead with your fabulousness. Plus, you'll feel better if you look like a million bucks.

"A good many dramatic situations begin with screaming."
—JANE FONDA,
ACTRESS AND ACTIVIST

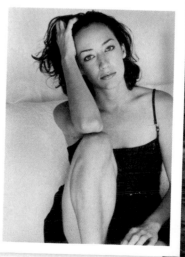

29

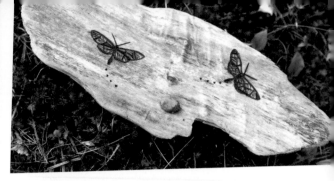

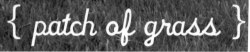

{ patch of grass }

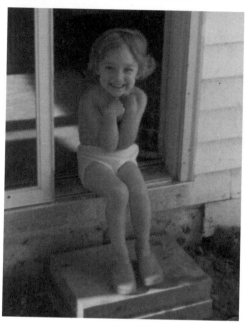

When I was growing up, my grandma was a surrogate mother to me. When Mom was busy putting herself through college (Vassar—she's a real brain) and bringing home the bacon from three jobs, my grandma filled in.

Until my dad and sister came into my life (a great two-fer!), I was an only child in rural Pawling, New York, with not much around besides dairy farms and hunting trailers. Grandma taught me that my imagination could be my best pal. "Look for the details," she'd tell me. We'd play fun games like "stare at the patch of grass." Whoever found the most detail would win a trip to the Red Rooster for chili dogs. She'd use words like gorgeous and delicious to describe all the beauty she saw. We'd spend hours sharing all the nooks and crannies of our dreams, exploring worlds with endless possibilities and wide-open spaces.

In 1978 our only TV was a little black-and-white eighteen-incher that we found at the dump. "Why would someone throw away a perfectly good television?" my grandmother would say in her thick, broken-English Colombian accent. The antennae were missing but she didn't care. Grandma was a crafty lady who constantly reinvented not only herself but everything we owned. I had no doubt that she would find a way to make the old TV work, perhaps with the metal hanger from the We

Care dry cleaners—also recovered from the dump. She scooped it up, and, with visions of Bugs Bunny racing through my head, off we zoomed in her old jalopy.

It wasn't until much later that I realized why someone threw out the TV Grandma said was meant for me. For my first seven years, I thought pink was the only color that television programs were transmitted in, which was fine by me because at the time pink was my favorite color (note the pink clogs). Grandma and I would spend hours in front of that TV imagining we were in Africa, riding elephants and swinging recklessly through jungle trees and cliffs just like Johnny Weissmuller did in those five-star Saturday-afternoon movies. We would don scarves and attitudes just like Katharine Hepburn in *The African Queen*. Grandma could make anything fun and adventurous. Anything but cancer.

So there I was, sitting in front of her, paralyzed with fear. "Grandma, ya know how I've

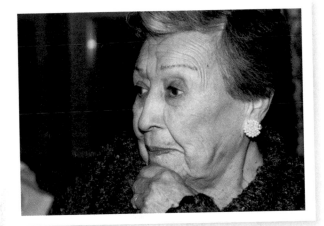

been at the doctor's a lot lately? Well, I have some bad news . . . I have cancer."

She took a long pause, mulled it over, then cleared her throat and said, "NO." Not *no* like *Oh God, say it isn't so*, no. *No* like *HELL NO, don't let anyone label you!*

In this way she was telling me to fight.

Not long after that my grandma passed away. My mom and I arrived at the hospital just in time for her to die in our arms. How I wished I could play one more game of "stare at the patch of grass" with her. Watching her die made death so real. But her last words said it all: "No" and "I love you"—words that made everything somehow seem more bearable. No matter what happened I was to be rebellious, buck the system, and know that she'd always be with me.

tip no.8

TELLING PEOPLE DOES
get easier over time

Your story won't turn on the waterworks (yours or theirs) each time you share it. It's like everything else: Distance and practice make the tough stuff manageable. It may sound strange, 'cause cancer isn't funny, but humor really helps. Most people will take their cues from you. If you deal with it well, so will they. People will take your lead. Talking about cancer in a candid way lets the elephant out of the room. Nobody knows how to start the conversation, what to ask, or how to act.

FAUX PAS!

Dear friends,
Don't ask me how long the doctors have given me! I mean, how gauche! If someone is so ill mannered, this would be my response (in fact it once was): "I don't know, how long have they given you, jackass?" That will stump them.

{ cancer humor }

Once the initial shock of my diagnosis wore off, my twisted sense of humor slithered out to terrorize once more. After all, I was the family clown, and this was great material. At times I was wildly inappropriate, making innocent bystanders deeply uncomfortable. Like when I told the CAT scan nurse that the barium sulfate suspension I was forced to drink (the creamy white fluid that makes your insides glow like a radioactive lava lamp) looked like the floor of a peep show. Bottoms up!

If I could laugh at my situation, I wouldn't drown in it. Though it did take time for them to get used to it, eventually my parents and friends became thankful for the levity I created by poking fun at the cancer. But be sensitive. Some people, including other cancer patients, just don't think cancer is something to make light of. So you really have to take the temperature of the room.

Also remember that humor walks a fine line. You can joke about cancer, but it gets tricky if other people do. Hearing "Hey sick chick, whas-sup tumor girl" on a bad day affects you in one of two ways: (1) You bust out laughing and slap the person on the back, thanking them for the ha-ha; (2) you get wildly offended and punch the person in the face as you open a can of ver-bal whoop-ass! Wannabe stand-up comics need to take the temperature of your room, too.

FAUX PAS!

Dear friends,
Don't pity me or tell me you know how I feel. (You don't and I don't expect you to!)

tip no.9

THE GAME OF
cancer telephone

Let's face it, getting diagnosed is just really good gossip. So you may want to make a pre-emptive strike before the word gets out. If the facts get muddled (as in a game of telephone), people will be sitting shivah in your living room while you're channel-surfing upstairs. My friend Erin Zammett Ruddy has a great gossip story.

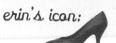
erin's icon:

PROFILE:
ERIN ZAMMETT RUDDY

AGE: 29

HAIR COLOR: Flaming red

EYES: Green

HEIGHT: 5'10" (that's what I used to write on my volleyball stat sheets . . . I think I'm more like 5'9½")

WEIGHT: Yeah, right!

HOMETOWN: Huntington, New York (Long Island, baby!)

OCCUPATION: Articles editor at *Glamour* magazine, blogger, author of *My (So-Called) Normal Life*

FAVORITE SAYING: "When life gives you lemons, make wine!"

BEST TIP: Go ahead and sweat the small stuff sometimes. It keeps your mind off sweating the big stuff . . . the stuff you can't always control.

Erin is one of the bitchin' Cancer Babes in my film. In fact, she's practically a cancerlebrity! Though the disease is something she may have to deal with for the rest of her life, Erin does not let cancer diminish her love for fashion, blogging, good food, great conversation, obsessing about her looks and weight, planning her future with her hubby, Nick, and running the show in her Jimmy Choo slingbacks. She's an articles editor at *Glamour* magazine, the author of *My (So-Called) Normal Life*, and a journalist, and speaks frequently at numerous cancer organizations including The Leukemia & Lymphoma Society and The G&P Foundation for Cancer Research. To Erin, cancer isn't about a diagnosis; it's about what you do with it.

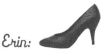
Erin:

My worst cancer experience (other than being diagnosed and having my sister be diagnosed) was hearing from my high school boyfriend that he'd "heard through the grapevine" I was dying. There is nothing I hate more than being part of the grapevine—especially when the news is about my health and is all wrong. I wasn't dying, I was eating a slice of pizza and watching *The Bachelor*, thank you very much. You never want to hear that you're dying but when you've just been diagnosed with cancer and you have no idea what your future holds, you *really* don't want to hear you're dying.

I've always hated the hometown gossip mill and really had to take it into consideration when I was diagnosed. I wanted to be sure I told friends myself before they heard it from their mothers who heard it from Mrs. So-and-So in the produce aisle of the grocery store. It's hard because someone getting cancer, as sad as it is, is good gossip, so of course people are going to be interested in spreading it. You just have to be sure you set the story straight as fast as possible.

I made a million calls and sent out a mass e-mail to my friends from high school. "I hope you're all sitting down," it began.

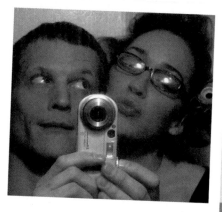

tip no. 10

DON'T GET *ambushed*

There's nothing worse than walking into a room full of people who all know about your diagnosis but you don't know that they know. My poor husband (then boyfriend), Brian, learned this the hard way. At the time, he was a big fancy writer/TV editor and he went to big fancy parties with TV people. The show he had just edited was nominated for an Emmy, so I was wildly proud and eager to help him celebrate. I figured my cancer diagnosis wasn't the topic of conversation around the watercooler, but I still wanted to make sure I wouldn't get those what-a-shame stares.

As the cab dashed us to the celebratory soiree, I softly chirped, "Honey do your co-workers know?"

"Know what?" he asked.

"Know that I have cancer." (Sometimes men are so obtuse.)

"Oh, that, yeah they all know, every last one of them. Each and every office boy and secretary in the whole joint knows!"

Okay, he didn't actually say this, but it's pretty much what I heard. It was too late for me to yell or cry or hide; we were already walking through the door blowing cheek kisses. I imagined everyone in the room writing me off as the sick chick. Brian and I don't fight in public; it's a rule. We play nice and then scrap at home. Which is exactly what happened later. I was paranoid and felt caught off guard and different. It was my crap, but unfortunately I blamed it on him.

Truth be told, it was a great night. I just dread the possibility of snoopy questions while I'm snacking on cheese, crackers, and passed hors d'oeuvres. That's a surefire recipe for the Heimlich maneuver! People don't mean to be abrasively direct, but sometimes questions fly out of their mouths without consideration for appropriate cocktail-speak. If you're not prepared with a few standard responses, something equally inappropriate might come out of yours.

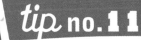

tip no.11

KEEP IN TOUCH
the easy way

Mass e-mails are an amazing way to avoid the exhaustion of telling the same story a zillion times. Crazy Sexy Cancer Updates are what I called mine. My cousin Suzanne's husband does a great mass e-mail after her every doctor visit. I love that he writes, "*We* just had *our* second scan." So sweet!

However, when writing, don't capitalize cancer. My friend Beth pointed out that I'd do that when I wrote her e-mails, and I realized that giving it so much importance is a no-no. So does saying "My cancer." Screw that. It's *the* cancer. In fact, spell it wrong: canser. It gives you power over that stupid little two-syllable word.

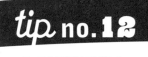

tip no.12

DON'T TELL
everyone

Yes, your world just changed forever, but don't go overboard spreading the word. In the beginning you may want to tell everyone, thinking you need all the support you can get. Still—some people are better off not knowing. For *your* sake.

Not long after the final diagnosis came in, my mom took me to a trendy spa for a pick-me-up beauty treatment. The welcome-to-our-fabulous-spa attendant handed me the client history form. I took one look at it and burst into tears. Shit! Just when I had forgotten about cancer for a nanosecond, bam! Why was "cancer" part of the checklist of allergies and conditions? Did I *have* to check off the cancer box? Why did *they* have to know?

I can understand the dentist, even the chiropractor, but the bikini waxer? I was there for some pubic maintenance, not a heart transplant! For people who aren't in the medical field, reading my disease, let alone pronouncing it, is a major event. And explaining it just opens up a huge can of worms. What, would they whip out some study on hot wax, vaginas, and vascular cancers? No, they'd be clueless and put on the gloves 'cause believe it or not, some people still think cancer is contagious. Plus, talking about the cancer while my helpless crotch follicles were being ripped out would only make the pain worse! My advice: Don't check the box if you're going for a bikini wax. Many medical professionals have assured me that you can keep your privacy during this kind of procedure.

a NEED-TO-KNOW *basis*

There are some friends and relatives you'll regret telling because they will never let you forget. You'll be at a family reunion and suddenly your aunt Sally (the bitter hypochondriac on your mother's side) will get that tender, fragile, concerned look on her face and in a made-for-television tampon-network way she'll ask some poor-you question like, "Sweetheart, how's your tragedy going today?" Huh? "Better after I stab you with my fork, Auntie dear." Even if you kick cancer's ass, that bitch will happily remind you that you'll always have to worry about it coming back. Don't take it personally; insensitive people usually have their own shit. Aunt Sally's probably still pissed that your mom got all the silver when their parents (God rest their souls) croaked. This has nothing to do with you, so just let it roll off your back as you poison her slab of casserole.

More people you should not tell: certain old colleagues. I recently ran into an old actor buddy—actually actor rival—of mine. Invariably it seemed to come down to one of us for a juicy part. Whoever pushed the other down the stairs first, won. I hadn't seen this woman since the news of my diagnosis had hit the audition circuit. She couldn't believe how good I looked (it totally stumped her); I couldn't believe how bad she looked.

We did that street-corner-catch-up-nutshell bullet-points thing. Mine was like, "I just got married, my movie is coming out, I signed a book deal, life is really great."

She didn't hear one word. "Do you still have your little problem," she asked in a whispered tone. "Is it all cleared up, gone far, far away?"

I have cancer, not some weird itchy yeast infection! "No, it's still around, but it's totally stable and I'm fine, happy even."

"Oh, well that's too bad. I'll pray for you." Huh?

This is what I hate, so let's make it a faux pas, some advice for noncancer people. Clip it out and send it anonymously to the biggest offenders!

FAUX PAS!

DON'T SAY THINGS LIKE:

> **You're so brave.**

> **You poor thing, I'll pray for you.**

> **Bless your tender heart.**

> **Whoa! You're fucked!**

What am I supposed to say?
Thank you?
Don't worry?
Are *you* okay?
Give me a break!

Then there are those passing acquaintances who don't really need to know because they don't really care, and telling them doesn't result in anything good for you: the dry cleaner, the deli guy, the exterminator, the mailman. One exception: I did tell my apartment building superintendent, whose pity came in handy for some overdue fix-its. Maybe it will bring me bad karma, but unless I greased this guy's wheel he was generally fairly lazy. Before cancer my air conditioner stayed in the window year-round, and the leak in my shower destroyed three sets of tiles *and* my Pottery Barn bath mat. After cancer I feebly (remember, I was an actress) put him to work! Technically, this is a good example of using the Cancer Card (see chapter 5).

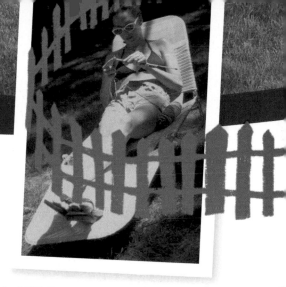

tip no.13

ESTABLISH *boundaries*

Some people and activities may have to take a back burner for now. When confronted with a social engagement or obligation,

ask yourself: Does it tire me or does it inspire me?

Stuff that brings ya down just has to go. Don't worry—your problems will still be around when this is over. If the people in your life can't roll with your decisions, then unfortunately the tribe has spoken, and they'll get kicked off Cancer Island. You'll find out pretty quickly who you can really count on not to take it personally. True colors appear like a neon sign.

Here's a juicy boundaries story. A few months after my diagnosis, a longtime friend of mine flew into town to take me to lunch. How nice, I thought. It had been awhile since I'd seen her, and I was touched by the effort. Well, about three sips into my soy latte, the following pamphlets appeared on the table:

FAUX PAS!

A Guide to End of Life Issues

Is Your Will in Order?

Who Pulls the Plug When This All Goes South?

Excuse me! I had barely let my (slow-moving) cancer settle in and now I probably wasn't going to make it through dessert. In fact, I'm surprised that my friend didn't have a hearse waiting outside. Major boundary citation!

Needless to say, cancer or not, all of us should have a will because we just don't know. But no one should force that shit on you. To this day I haven't done my will, out of spite. But now that I'm married and have a house, I have to get over myself and do it. I mean, it is the mature thing, right? Perhaps next week . . . maybe. Nah!

Dear friends and acquaintances,
Don't try to bond with me by telling me you know someone with cancer, too, and they just died! It won't bring us close.

When I shared this tidbit with my mom, she told me that she hears this as well—and it's always painful. What are these people thinking? Were they raised in a barn? Hello, earth to healthy obtuse person. In case you didn't know, death is a touchy topic to both cancer patients and their families. Major faux pas!

Don't be surprised if you find yourself comforting your friends when they process your news—you may need to set boundaries around that as well. I was amazed at how many people needed me to make them feel better! Once the death-reminder button gets pushed, everyone freaks, not just you. I let a lot of people cry on my shoulder in the beginning, and it was really weird and exhausting. One friend—let's call her Bernice—burst into tears and drooled all over my favorite camel-colored cashmere sweater, "Why you, why you? If this could happen to you it could happen to me! Oh, dear God! Life is so unfair!" I haven't heard from Bernice since (good riddance). If you find

yourself comforting others far too often, stop, drop, and roll! Steer clear of the emotional vampires who make it all about themselves. They'll just zap your energy while you're trying to get your feet on the ground.

In fact, this may be time for a little house-cleaning, and I don't mean with the mop and broom (although a tidy space does create a good healing vibe). I mean your social life. It's time to renovate the little black book. You just don't have enough energy to tap yourself out. That's the old you. If you're like me, you deal with everyone else's needs but your own. The people who really matter will step up to the plate. To the rest: au revoir, adios, beat it!

tip no. 14

FIND A
pen pal

Writing is a great way to share your cancer conundrums, and who better to share it with than a gal going through the same or similar? For some of you, finding a pen pal with a matching cancer will be a piece of cake. But for us ladies with the rare cancers, it can be more challenging. I generally hold my breath as I travel down the official lists of popular cancers from organizations such as the National Cancer Institute (NCI) or the American Medical Association (AMA). I wonder, *Will mine be on it? Will it stop at vagina and never make it to vascular?*

My first pal was a big gong! I did a Google search and found her on the Internet, and unfortunately cyberspace is where I should have left her. For the sake of her anonymity (and my safety), let's call her Helga. Helga had an amaz-

ing story. Not only did she have the same cancer as me, she apparently had cured herself of it naturally. What?! I was looking under every holistic rock for the miracle elixir and, wow, was I psyched to find her. There was just one problem: Helga was a born-again, and her idea of writing me inspirational letters chock-full of experience and advice went something like this: YOU'RE SCREWED! CONVERT, CONVERT! MY JESUS OR ELSE!

Sadly, I was never able to glean any nutritional nuggets through her cacophony of spiritual threats. She petrified me! I was so busy dodging Jesus bullets that I didn't have time to think or defend myself. So I'm not the most (structured) religious type, but I'm certainly not a hedonistic God-hater. Do I pray? Yes. Is it always to God? No. Sometimes it's to Buddha or Elvis or other peeps I'll share with you in chapter 4. Some people might make you feel like you have to be this enlightened spiritual person now that cancer has shown you the light. Bullshit. Yes, it's a wake-up call, but does that mean you need to come into the fold? Hell no! Cancer isn't gonna take you out just because you're chatting with the "wrong" Godhead. Needless to say, I told Helga that Satan was my homeboy and changed my e-mail.

That experience almost had me calling it quits on the whole pen pal thing, and then my doctor connected me with Paula. Paula makes me laugh, and she gets the whole living-with-cancer trip in a way no one else in my posse does. For us it's not about getting it out and getting it over, it's about the big picture, long haul. She gets it 'cause she lives it just like me. Some cancer peeps call their oncologist if they sneeze. I don't. I've never called him once, even though there have been a few times when I've wondered *Is this pain from my period or do I suddenly have a cancerous cantaloupe dangling from my fallopian tube?*

Cancer paranoia is pretty common.

Will a simple ache ever be benign again? It depends on how imaginative you are! I'm twisted, so half the time I'm a day away from the ICU. These are the times I write Paula. "Does this stuff happen to you?" She has put my mind to ease on several occasions and made me realize that some of my fears are silly and some are real, and I should be responsible and look into them. She also keeps me on track with my checkups because (and this may sound irresponsible but at least I'm honest) I am notorious for blowing them off. I've never seen a picture of Paula or even heard her voice, but she is a big player on my cancer team. My coach.

Find your Paula—if she's as cool as mine, she'll make the whole experience easier. Just ask your doctor for recommendations before delving into cyberspace. They have access to people who share the same challenges as you—and docs can prescreen them, so to speak, for sanity.

chapter two in review:

remember:

Even if it's just for a few hours, find a way to take a mental vacation from cancer.

Create a space that's all your own.

Give yourself time to process the diagnosis and let it sink in.

Most people will take their cues from you. If you deal with it well, so will they.

Steer clear of the emotional vampires that make your cancer all about themselves.

Don't take part in activities that don't make you feel good.

Surround yourself with people you love.

Find a simpatico pen pal.

Don't let the bastards get you down.

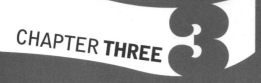

cancer COLLEGE

Make no mistake—cancer makes you very busy! In the beginning, the phone rings off the hook, well-meaning friends fill your inbox with statistics and research, the major cancer hospitals find their way into your Rolodex, and legions of cancer books infiltrate your bookshelves like soldiers heading to the front lines in phalanx formation. Good-bye

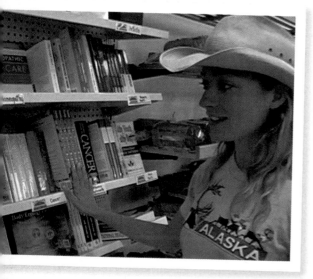

Catcher in the Rye, hello *A Cancer Battle Plan* (which is actually a very good book). I don't care what you majored in or flunked out of, your new profession is getting well. If you've never run a business before, then this is the perfect time to learn. By the time we're through, you'll be the Warren Buffett of Cancer Management.

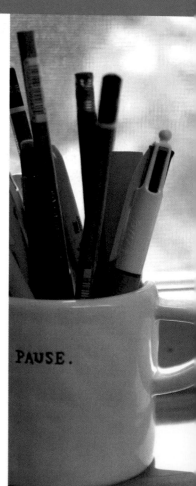

PAUSE.

Welcome to Cancer College, freshman year. Visitor maps and a tour of the campus happen on the hour. If you're interested, please meet at the vitals room. Also, in case you didn't come prepared (understandable, since this all happened very quickly: One minute you're buying a bucket of wings at KFC, next minute bam! Ivy League cancer school), Trapper Keepers and pocket protectors are available at the campus bookstore along with chemo barf bags and heating pads. (P.S.: Heating pads can be used to reduce the pain around your IV site.)

You're currently enrolled in our most popular crash course: *Help, I Have to Organize My Badass Cancer Self!* Not to worry. Consider me your resident assistant. I'm happy to answer any questions and show you the ropes. You'll be spending a good portion of your time at the campus library, studying subjects like Your Cancer Body, Yourself. I encourage you to familiarize yourself with your afflicted organ/organs. Makes sense, right? The knowledge may come in handy, especially if your doctor decides that one of your organs is disposable. Wouldn't you at least like to know what it did before it no longer does it?

In the sophomore lounge you will socialize with patients who are slightly more experienced than you. Be warned: They may bully you because you're the new kid on the block. Hold your ground. Just because they've had cancer longer doesn't give them alpha dog status. You are just as entitled to your dramas as they are. And don't get into the staging game! Stage IV patients are no more superior than Stage I. Please!

Then there's the cafeteria (more on that in chapter 6). You will be eating mostly organic this semester and cutting back on the white crap—it makes you fat and unhappy and anyway, don't you already have enough to deal with? It'll be tough at first, but we at the university find that size 6 jeans and an immunity boost are good motivators.

Okay, we don't mean to overwhelm you, but there is one more thing. You see, here at the Harvard of Healing, your education is one part learning and one part doing. Why wait until graduation to put your new skills into action? Do what the Google boys did and launch your healing start-up (let's call it "Save My Ass Technologies, Inc.") right from your dorm room. Granted, things may be rocky at first, but before you know it you'll be featured in *Fortunate* magazine and your stock will be busting through the roof!

What's cancer anyway?

To truly answer that question, let's start with what cancer is not.

Cancer isn't a punishment you deserve based on your actions or lack thereof.

Cancer isn't a disgrace caused by a crazy drug-induced sexcapade. Cancer isn't a curse passed down through generations of misbehaved families who robbed banks, drank too much, and forgot to send thank-you notes.

There is nothing taboo about cancer, and it certainly isn't contagious.

You won't turn green if you share my straw, and there's no need to reach for the surgical mask when you see me approach.

Some people are very superstitious when it comes to talking openly about the disease, as if words themselves carry potential harm. Rest assured: Cancer chitchat will not leave you vulnerable to the same voodoo-chicken-claw magic that strikes down innocent bystanders who accidentally walk under ladders or open umbrellas indoors.

Often cancer patients are made to feel it's socially inappropriate to be cancer patients. We're expected to file the reality away in some far-off emotional safe so that other people can enjoy their fresh pea soup in peace. People's body language reveals a lot about our society's preconceived prejudices about cancer. It happens to all of us. Watch as one of your friends slowly backs away as you reveal your scarlet letter C. Take it with a grain of salt. Nobody wants to die; it's just too permanent.

tip no. 15

EVERYBODY HAS A THEORY.
listen to what resonates.

Much has been written about the psychology of cancer—the cancer profile or personality. In Chinese medicine the lungs represent grief; the liver, anger. Since these are the two areas where my tumors established residence, I became very interested in exploring the idea that somehow by not expressing those feelings properly, I was to blame for my illness. Yes, I'm sad about a lot of things, and pissed off, too. But fuck that!

I remember one newbie healer type telling me that "my" cancer was karmic and that I had mountains of bad stuff to dig my way through. Don't get me wrong, I have great respect for alternative medicine, but you have to find the jewels among the woo-woo crystals. Like I have time to deal with my ancestors' dramas? Give me a break! Anyone can print HEALER on a business card. Just because you took a two-day Shaman 101 workshop (with breakout sessions) at the Milwaukee "open center" doesn't mean you have any business treating people. Folks like that could really benefit from a class called Cancer for a Day. They'd crap their purple-colored chakra pants and think twice before dumping half-baked notions on patients who need support.

{ cancer: the basics }

Now that we know what cancer isn't, we can explore what cancer is. Most of us think of cancer as a disease characterized by the runaway growth of cells due to a genetic mutation. While this is basically true, it's only part of the picture. As my doctor describes it, cancer is actually the result of an imbalance between cell growth and cell death. All of our cells have a life span, and inside each cell is a code that tells it when to call it quits. This is called programmed cell death. Besides that, each cell has genes whose specific job is to look out for mutations in the genetic code. When a mutation is recognized, the cell automatically destroys itself. It knows it's a bad apple and takes one for the team.

For cancer to happen, then, there has to be a mutation that damages the policing gene. In this case the bad cells continue to replicate (and refuse to kick the bucket)—to the point that they begin to choke out the good guys.

If this is all too technical, here's another way to think about it. Did you ever see that Michael Keaton box-office flop *Multiplicity*? Each clone that Michael Keaton made of himself got weirder and less functional, to the point that one of the copies was a drooling idiot. Of course, in a movie this makes for big wackiness and hijinks. But in your body, too many crazies running amok can be deadly serious.

43

INCURABLE ISN'T A DECLARATION,
it's a dare!

As I mentioned, when I was first diagnosed I heard lots of outrageous you-gotta-be-kidding-me blah blah blah. I had a choice: Curl up and suck my thumb or toss my ass out of bed and do something! It wasn't long before I realized that I would have to take charge of my own health care.

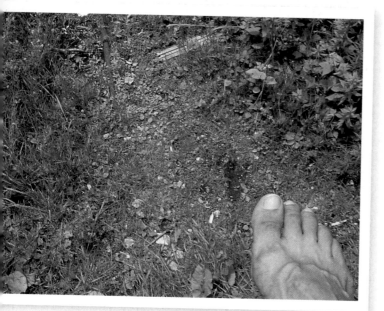

On one of many post-diagnosis gloomy afternoons, I was overmedicating at Starbucks and feeling sorry for myself. There I was, slumped over in the window, watching the problemless perfect people gleefully skip on by. I was nurturing a fantasy of one last toxic blowout—a dirty, drug-fueled "good-bye life!" super-disco. The who's who of the party crowd would all be there, and they'd actually pay attention to me. We'd dance and grind inap-

propriately till the undertaker came to collect me for my nonrefundable dirt nap. Just then an angel (well, actually it was a pigeon) wildly flapped its wings, as if commanding me to look for the source of its agitation. That's when I saw it. There in front of me was a magnificent billboard with the coolest ad I'd ever seen. It had soccer hottie David Beckham screaming like a testosterone-filled gladiator, and it said: "Impossible is just a big word thrown around by small men who find it easier to live in the world they've been given, than to explore the power they have to change it. Impossible is an opinion, not a fact. Impossible isn't a declaration, it's a dare. Impossible is potential. Impossible is temporary. Impossible is nothing." Amen! I immediately replaced the word *impossible* with *incurable*, and it helped me cultivate some of my own inner testosterone.

Some of you may have been stamped with an expiration date that just doesn't jive with your future plans. Like an old carton of milk in the back of the fridge, you've been told that your days on the shelf are numbered. If I were your angel, I would remind you that nobody can predict the future. Don't be gunned down by what you hear. It's just information. It's not impossible.

GRAND OPENING!

SAVE MY ASS
TECHNOLOGIES, INC.

Getting organized and setting clear goals will help you establish your direction. Since you certainly have a lot on your plate, it's important to devise a strategy for success. Is Bill Gates wishy-washy? What about Oprah Winfrey? Does she say stuff like *I can't decide* or *Whatever you think is best*? No. When they say jump, their staffs crack their heads on the ceiling. While Gates and Winfrey don't have cancer, use them as a business model and make recovery your ultimate goal.

Below you will learn some basic managerial skills that will help you on your road to recovery. If you've never been the go-get-'em aggressive type, thank cancer for the opportunity. As my lovely (yet annoyingly blunt) shrink says, "It's time to grow up and show up."

Every effective CEO knows the key to success is employing a staff of winners. Your very first job as CEO of a cancer recovery conglomerate is to handpick a save-my-ass staff of family, friends, doctors, and/or other kinds of healers. Only the cream of the crop will do.

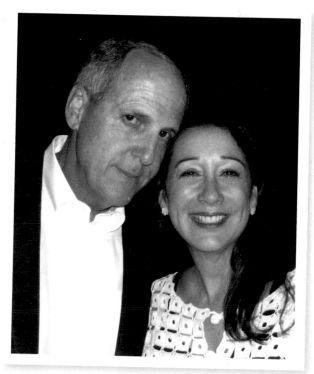

tip no. **17**

TAKE A LITTLE
cancer roadtrip

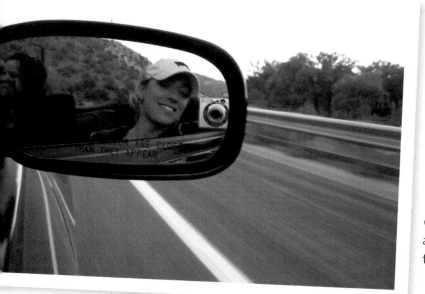

Sometimes you have to be willing to go the extra mile to find the right doctor. A study published in the September 2003 *Journal of the National Cancer Institute* found that "patients who traveled 15 or more miles for their care had one-third the risk of death of those living closer. Moreover, for every 10 miles that a patient traveled for care, the risk of death decreased by 3.2%."

What does this mean? For starters, the quality of care out there varies greatly, so you may benefit from looking beyond your town or state. You may even consider going out of the country. It also proves that people with a proactive attitude simply have a better chance of kicking ass!

SKYWISH

Delta Air Lines and United Way have joined forces to form SkyWish, a program that uses frequent flier miles donated by Delta's frequent fliers to transport patients—cancer patients included—to medical treatment. To apply for flight tickets, contact your local United Way or United Way of America at (800) UWA-2757, extension 285.

tip no.18

WHEN DOCTOR SHOPPING,
REMEMBER THAT SICKNESS IS BIG BUSINESS—
don't get sucked in

Not every doctor you visit is going to be a perfect match. No hard feelings, but if the shoe doesn't fit, keep shopping—preferably at Prada. This isn't a time to cut cancer coupons and buy cheap. Quality lasts and you want to, too. Listen to your gut. Go with the team that feels right.

Think of all the doctors, nurses, healers, and helpers as part of your workforce, and remember that healing takes place on multiple levels. Many factors contribute to a diagnosis; some are in our control, others are not. Be open, stretch yourself, and try new things. You may need to balance common Western theories with some additional alternative therapies. Have you ever done acupuncture?

What about energy work or massage? Are you sweating enough? Think of healing as a whole-body experience. Sometimes treating the symptom just isn't enough (again, more on this in chapter 6).

Picture yourself as a chair with four legs: emotional, spiritual, physical, and mental. If just one leg becomes wobbly, you're more likely to topple over. I'm not suggesting that you become a full-time healing junkie or weekend workshop warrior (unless that makes you happy). Take it all in stride, but be curious. Also remember that there are a lot of quacks hanging out CURE FOR CANCER IN JUST THREE EASY PAYMENTS OF $19.95 signs. Do your research.

tip no.19

SEEK SECOND (AND THIRD!)
opinions

It's true that you shouldn't judge a book by its cover, but you can tell a lot by a waiting room. The second hospital I went to, Medical Center XX (name withheld for reasons having to do with the law and my bank account), had stiff wooden chairs, dirty carpets, and a Scotch-Taped sign that read: ABSOLUTELY NO FOOD OR DRINK. There were no dynamic new wings named after rich benefactors or perky young candy stripers pushing carts with secondhand romance novels to brighten your day.

The nurse in reception intimidated me more than the cancer. No Hello. No Welcome! No I'm sorry you have to go through this, dear. Only nastiness and a lot of it. It baffles me when disgruntled life-haters get jobs at cancer hospitals. Shouldn't there be some sort of personality screening test? Example: "When cancer patients are struggling to find their insurance card, you (1) tell them not to worry and to take their time; (2) ask if you can help; or (3) tell them that their blind ass needs to figure it out 'cause they're holdin' up the line!"

Take Nurse Ratchet, the Cruella du jour. She was a portly drill sergeant with tropical-scene nail tips that clacked furiously on her IBM PC. I sat nervous and confused as she barked orders in her thick accent. She wasn't registering me for my appointment; she was hazing me for irresponsibly getting sick. Like I could have prevented it by wearing a hat and scarf or, for God's sake, not leaving the house with wet hair!

"KRISTIN CARR?" she snapped.

"YES MA'AM!"

"FILL OUT THESE THOUSAND FORMS AND DON'T MAKE ME USE THE WITE-OUT! DO YOU HAVE A CATHETER?"

"NO MA'AM!"

"DO YOU HAVE A PORT OR A STENT?" I paused, looking confused. What did that mean? Was it something I was supposed to pick up on my way? I was starting to feel beads of perspiration pooling in my armpits. "HELLLOOOOO! A PORT, A STENT, A DAGGER IN YOUR HEART? A SPEAR THROUGH YOUR CHEST? A NAIL ON YOUR CROSS?"

"NOOOOO!" I howled.

"Give your insurance card to Maria in 307 and don't forget to give me back my pen."

After I was released from Maria in 307, I found my way back to my parents. My mom had a concerned look on her face. "Where are all the mink coats?" she innocently whispered. What she really meant was: Where are all the rich people? PC or not, when you're sick there's something comforting about walking into a plush waiting room filled with well-dressed rich folks. But as I was soon to find out, when it comes to finding the best available cancer treatment, hobnobbing with the A-list cancer crowd is not always where it's at.

If Medical Center XX was the rusted-out Chevette of cancer hospitals, then YY Health Center was a Bentley. This place was four-star. Its luxurious leather sofas, waterfalls, and beautiful chemo suites made me feel like I was checking into a fancy spa. They even gave out free upscale snacks, like shortbreads, lattes, and bottled springwater. And the wide-grinned, Stepford-style nurses were accessorized like perky waitresses with flare buttons that read: NEED A HUG? Why yes I do, squeeze away!

So far, so good, I thought. I could be comfortable here, could even catch up on months of unanswered e-mails in the free high-speed Internet lounge. Yet three hours later I was no longer amused. Four hours later I was irate! The famous doctor (let's call him Dr. Richards, or DICK for short) finally called my name. Never once did he apologize for keeping us waiting. He just sat there, smugly spouting treatment options that "probably wouldn't work anyway."

When we asked a few questions based on some of our research, he seemed amused. What pedestrians! After a few minutes the appointment was over and so were his chances of working with me. His God complex was so déclassé! To him I was a walking statistic; to me Dr. Dick was a jerk who needed a good ol'-fashioned spatula spanking, just like Grandma used to give. No hard feelings, but sorry, Dr. Dick, you're underqualified. Next!

the PITFALLS of getting only one opinion

I met my friend Terri through an ex-boyfriend about thirteen years ago. Sometimes you don't know what a relationship is ultimately meant to give you. In this case it was a marvelous friendship with a brilliant woman. Terri was my first friend to be diagnosed with cancer, but unfortunately she wouldn't be my last.

terri's icon:

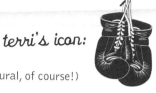

AGE: 40-something-ish

HAIR COLOR: Blond (natural, of course!)

EYES: Blue

HEIGHT: 5'4"

WEIGHT: 120 and, according to my husband, just right!

HOMETOWN: Maywood, New Jersey, affectionately referred to as Mayberry by its bored teen citizenry

OCCUPATION: Licensed psychotherapist; television acting teacher at Stone Street Studios and Tisch School of the Arts at New York University; co-host of the talk show "On Your Mind—Mental Health and Healing"; and currently training to be a kickboxing instructor!

FAVORITE SAYING: "You are either part of the problem or part of the solution."

BEST TIP: When we travel together, my childhood pals and I have a ritual. As soon as we hit the highway, we open all the windows and scream at the top of our lungs. My tip is to scream often: It's very cathartic!

She's the person I turn to with the hard stuff. No matter what advice she gives, she always delivers it in a way that makes me put things in perspective and cackle about being human. Here's what she has to say about the importance of second opinions:

Terri:

My first surgeon at ZZ Medical Institute (name withheld for the usual reasons) took out half of my thyroid. He didn't call me in the ten days before my follow-up, so I thought all was well. When I showed up for the appointment, he informed me that he hadn't even looked at the pathol-

ogy yet! I thought, Wow, that's weird. How 'bout you look at it now! So he looked and said, "Oh well. It's malignant."

Being a cancer virgin, I said, "Is that the bad one?"

"No, it's such a low-grade cancer, I wouldn't even call it cancer," he said.

Well, you can call it a chair, but that doesn't really make it one, now, does it? So I did a ton of research and found out that it wasn't so low-grade, that it could move to my lungs and bones, and that the tumor was the size of a plum. When I saw him again, I told him that I was concerned about the other side of my

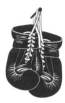

thyroid, but he was adamant that there was nothing wrong with it and that basically I was hysterical. "But what if you're wrong!" I said.

"Well, I would be very sorry, and you would be very, very sorry."

To which I responded, "I'm not worried about being sorry, I'm worried about being dead. And you being sorry while shooting nine holes in Westches-ter gives me no comfort!" I fired him that day. Turned out he was wrong and there was cancer on the other side of my thyroid—two different kinds of very rare cancer. Six months later, I had to redo the surgery.

Lesson learned: You and you alone are responsible for your health. Don't pick a doctor out of fear and don't assume they're all equal. I did and was sorry.

tip no.**20**

HUNT FOR THE TOP TACO, *the big banana*

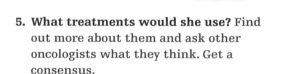

Don't sign up with the first doctor you meet. Even if you feel totally confident in that first doctor, shop around so that you are absolutely sure. Here's a quick qualifications crib sheet:

1. **Look for the diploma on the wall.** It should come from a country you can identify, and preferably not an island in the Caribbean.

2. **Can he pronounce the name of your cancer?** If so, can he do it five times really fast?

3. **How many patients with your disease has she treated** since cadaver class in '82?

4. **Is he a specialist?** A researcher? Specialists have more expertise than general oncologists and are more likely to be up to speed on the leading, most cutting-edge treatments. If your doctor is a researcher and has been published, obtain copies of his articles. They will give you insight into the treatment strategies he embraces.

5. **What treatments would she use?** Find out more about them and ask other oncologists what they think. Get a consensus.

6. **Does he have the bedside manner** of Dog the Bounty Hunter?

7. **What kind of reputation** does she have in the medical community?

Find the person who knows the most about your disease. Four opinions later, I chose to work with Dr. George Demetri, the director of the Sarcoma Department at the Dana-Farber Cancer Institute. Good-bye Chevettes and Bentleys, hello vintage cherry-red '66 Mustang! I knew that if the shit hit the fan, Dana-Farber would be the place for me.

Dr. Demetri is a scientist and a researcher. He's not just reading about the new stuff; he's

THE TOP 10 *cancer hospitals*

U.S. News & World Report publishes an annual list of the top fifty hospitals in the nation for cancer research and treatment. The top ten for 2006 are listed below. Many are the founding facilities for medical breakthroughs in cancer.

1. **Memorial Sloan-Kettering, New York.** Memorial Sloan-Kettering is a not-for-profit hospital. It's also an NCI-designated Cancer Center, which means it receives funding from the National Cancer Institute for things like research resources and access to state-of-the-art technologies. www.mskcc.org

2. **University of Texas M. D. Anderson Cancer Center, Houston.** M.D. Anderson has earned an international reputation for scientific excellence and outstanding research-driven cancer care. www.mdanderson.org

3. **Johns Hopkins Hospital, Baltimore.** Recognized worldwide for advances in cancer research and treatment. www.hopkinskimmelcancercenter.org

4. **Mayo Clinic, Rochester, Minnesota.** The Mayo Clinic is considered one of the best when it comes to patient satisfaction. It's centered in Minnesota, but clinics are also available in Florida and Arizona. www.mayoclinic.org

5. **Dana-Farber Cancer Institute, Boston.** Rated number five in the country—and number one in New England. www.dana-farber.org

6. **University of Washington Medical Center, Seattle.** An outstanding cancer hospital that treats cancers common and rare, and offers consultation, diagnosis, treatment, and follow-up care. www.uwmedicine.org

7. **Duke University Medical Center, Durham, North Carolina.** Located on the campus of Duke University, this is the youngest of the top cancer centers on this list. Don't let its infancy fool you: Duke's clinical and research programs rival the best. www.cancer.duke.edu

8. **University of Chicago Hospitals, Illinois.** Also an NCI-designated Cancer Center, the University of Chicago Hospitals cancer program is consistently ranked high for its advanced treatment methods and team of top professionals. www.uchospitals.edu/specialties/cancer/

9. **UCLA Medical Center, Los Angeles.** UCLA's claim to fame was making the first diagnosis of the AIDS virus. The cancer research is award winning. UCLA has made the list fifteen consecutive years. www.cancer.mednet.ucla.edu

10. **University of California–San Francisco Medical Center.** One of a handful of Comprehensive Cancer Centers in the state of California—a designation that recognizes success at combining innovative research and cutting-edge patient care. http://cancer.ucsf.edu

on the forefront of developing it. Dr. D has kind eyes, a nice smile, and a million-dollar brain. I should have had the same standards for some of my loser boyfriends! Every known factoid about my disease is embedded in his temporal lobe (smart brain word). And though he shoots from the hip, he does it in a compassionate way. Best of all, he respects me as much as I respect him. He calls my family Team Carr and is always happy to spend extra time explaining stuff so that I understand it. Most importantly, Dr. D gets straight to the point when delivering my news—no dillydally dispatch. There's nothing worse than sitting through small talk about the weather when your results are burning a hole through a manila folder.

Thankfully, there is a new wave of oncologists out there who've reevaluated the shock-and-awe "war on cancer" approach of the 1970s and '80s. Back then, the common goal was to shrink the tumors at any cost, and as a result many people suffered tremendously. Often the patient's quality of life was completely destroyed—only to have the cancer return.

Today, in many cases (such as my own) the goal is stability, not shrinkage. Understandably, people can get blown away by a cancer diagnosis; sometimes they then give up too soon or allow the disease to rule their lives in a debilitating way. Most people don't think about diseases like high blood pressure or diabetes in the same way that they think about cancer, and yet much of what doctors are doing today is treating cancer like a kind of chronic disease. Perhaps we need to stop "waging war" and start understanding, so that cancer will seem less threatening both physically and mentally and people will be able to live many years with the disease . . . if they have to.

tip no.21

IT TAKES A VILLAGE,
so create your tribe and delegate!

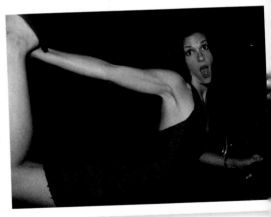

My hilarious (and flexible) sister Leslie

Assign tasks. Enlist your family and friends for support. For instance, let someone else do the Googling. I asked my best friend Lisa to be my research queen. She cut through the junk and sent me only what I needed to know. I didn't want the graphic details about what would happen if the EHE spread to my testicles. Also, who the hell wants to read grim stats? Way to wreck the party! "Sorry, gotta run; I'm told I'll be kicking the bucket in about forty-five minutes, so I'll have to pass on that second Cosmo."

My tribe played essential roles. In the beginning Dad was my navigator, getting me to all my appointments painfully early "just to play it safe." This was crucial, as I've inherited my mom's sense of direction, which means left equals right and west is east. Fine for a scenic country drive, but mega-stressful on scan day. Hospitals sometimes make you wait months

EMOTIONAL PILEUP ON
THE INFORMATION SUPERHIGHWAY

Erin:

Cancer should come with a warning: DO NOT GOOGLE ME. Ever the dependable informant, Google will present you with a ton of information about your cancer. But beware: Some of it is sure to be overwhelming, confusing, and downright scary, especially for a cancer newbie. If you're too fragile to navigate the Google maze, have someone else do it for you!

for just a few minutes with the Top Taco, so don't be tardy!

Mom became my cancer secretary, keeping track of the endless paperwork and insurance claims that seem to reproduce like rats in a city subway. My sister was my comic relief. Some patients like a calm, serious atmosphere surrounding their hospital visits. Not me. I like a full-on goat rodeo. Leslie has an endless supply of inappropriate jokes and a fascination with medical supply closets bearing yellow BIOHAZARD stickers. Needless to say, there's never a dull moment. During one memorable

visit, she got her hands on some rubber gloves and a tube of K-Y jelly. Need I say more? We all burst into hysterics as the words "bend over" echoed through the nurses' station.

Ask yourself who can lighten your load. Maybe you need help with the kids, someone to pick up your dry cleaning or do some wash? Or perhaps a nice home-cooked meal would take the pressure off. The people who love you will be happy to donate their time. Sometimes making your day a little easier is the best gift a person can give.

tip no.22

CREATE AND MAINTAIN
a medical binder

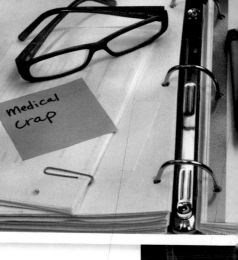

Information and medical documents will be flying around faster than thirty-something fashionistas at a Manolo Blahnik sample sale. Now, I'm a Virgo (translation: totally anal and obsessive). My mom is an Aries (translation: totally organized and proactive). Together (well, actually, it was mostly her) we created a bitchin' medical binder, complete with every scrap of cancer information I had. Here are some basic steps to get you started:

- **Be practical and thorough,** but have fun, too. Make it a scrapbook if you want; add journals, pictures, articles, or quotes that inspire you.

- **It's important to write down your questions before your appointments,** and refer to them during your visit. Make sure you understand what the doctors are telling you. Even if they make you feel like the information they're imparting is simple and easy to comprehend, make them explain it yet again if it isn't crystal clear. Be redundant, slow, impaired—who cares! Don't be intimidated by their elliptical medical jargon. Lots of doctors come from a far-off land where translators rarely make it out alive. If you can't find someone to go with you to appointments and be your scribe, then take a tape recorder so you don't have to worry about missing something in the haze of all that doctor-speak.

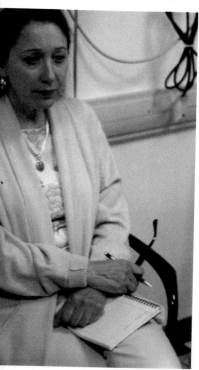

- **Keep track of all the treatments** you receive, as well as your medications and their dosages (including herbal supplements and vitamins). Be sure to list their side effects.

- **Record when you go** to the hospital and for what reason.

- **Write a detailed summary** of your appointment or hospital stay. You never know when you'll need to remember the specifics.

- **Create a calendar planner** to keep track of appointments and medication refills.

- **Include a section** for important phone numbers, addresses, and business cards. If your hospital gives you a registration card, you can safely store it here.

- **Make copies of your insurance information** so you can easily supply it when needed.

- **Keep extra paper** in your binder for note taking.

- **Collect maps of the local area** around your hospital, including some good restaurant choices—especially those with takeout! Cafeteria food sucks. You need a backup plan.

You can also order premade binders that can be further customized from www.cancer 101.org, the Lance Armstrong foundation (livestrong.org), or my Web site at www .crazysexycancer.com. Go ahead, take my mom home; just return her before the holidays.

This is one of the most important organizational tips in this book, so make or buy your binder posthaste!

> "Love is what we were born with. Fear is what we learned here."
> — **MARIANNE WILLIAMSON,**
> **AUTHOR AND LECTURER**

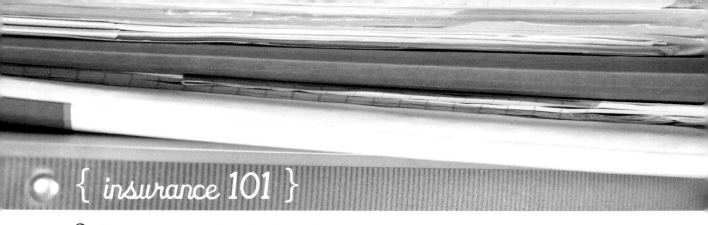

Beating cancer comes with a price tag. Sad, but true. So it's vital that you understand what type of insurance you have. And if you aren't covered, you must be aware of what your options are. If this section makes your eyes glaze over, you're not alone. Getting up to speed on insurance matters is a total drag, but this stuff is important to figure out, so pace yourself and read it in small doses if you have to.

tip no.23

LEARN WHAT YOUR COVERAGE INCLUDES
before beginning treatment

You might be responsible for payment of fees and services if you don't follow your insurance plan's guidelines. Here's a list of questions you should ask of your insurer before beginning treatment:

- **Is preauthorization required** for any prescribed surgical procedures or treatments? If so, ask your doctor for the "CPT codes." Armed with those, you'll be able to find out from your insurance company if the treatments is covered. If it isn't, you can appeal. Ask your doctor to explain why the heck the procedure is necessary.

- **Does your coverage have any exclusions**—items or services for which benefits are not provided? For example, some plans that cover cancer therapy don't cover the expensive growth factors often required to replace blood cells depleted by chemotherapy.

- **Are second opinions covered?** Or are they required for certain procedures, such as surgery?

- **If you are covered by an indemnity plan** (aka fee-for-service plan), what are the amounts of your yearly deductible and the percentage of your co-payment (usually 20 percent)? Cancer therapy is expensive, so you also should find out whether your plan has a maximum out-of-pocket expenditure per calendar year. In some plans, once a patient has paid $3,000 in deductibles and co-payments, the insurance plan provides full coverage of the remaining balance.

and how will you be paying for your treatment today, MISS SASSY PANTS?

Here are two typical billing procedures.

At a hospital, clinic, or hospital-affiliated doctor's office: If any member of your health care team is in practice within a hospital, the hospital's billing department will usually bill your insurance company directly and then bill you for any balance due.

At a private doctor's or specialist's office: Some private doctors or specialists will bill your insurance company; others require payment from you when services are rendered. If you pay the doctor, you are responsible for sending the receipt to your insurance company for reimbursement.

tip no.24

MAX OUT your insurance

Many cancer patients don't take full advantage of their insurance plans because they don't know about a benefit, they're confused, or they're put off by the paperwork. Some of your claims may be turned down or reimbursed at a reduced level. There are many reasons for claim rejection. However, you can appeal a refused claim or a reduced payment. If you need help filing a claim and your friends and family can't assist, ask a social worker for help. Private companies and some community organizations also offer help with filing insurance claims.

"your policy does NOT COVER this procedure"

If you receive the news that "your policy does not cover this procedure," you have the right to see that policy language in writing. Make sure these policy restrictions were in place when your coverage started. Otherwise you may have the right to coverage under the insurance laws of your state. To locate a copy of insurance laws online, go to www.health insuranceinfo.net. This site will let you view a *Getting and Keeping Health Insurance* booklet for every state and the District of Columbia. It also provides phone numbers for each state's insurance department.

> "The question isn't who is going to let me; it's who is going to stop me."
> —AYN RAND, AUTHOR

56

GET SOMEONE
on your case

If you find that you're constantly butting heads with your insurance company, you may want to inquire about case management. Most insurance companies have case managers, often registered nurses, who act as liaisons between you and the company and help coordinate payments to your health care providers.

If your insurance company doesn't have case managers or your claims continue to be denied, you do have another option: the Patient Advocate Foundation. The PAF acts as a liaison among patients, insurers, employers, and creditors. The foundation frequently deals with denied access to clinical trials or home health care, as well as with restrictions on payments for prescription drugs. Access the PAF online at www.patientadvocate.org.

{ not insured? }

It may be worthwhile to investigate other sources of financial aid if you aren't covered by an insurance plan. It's difficult to get an insurance company to underwrite you for a new policy if you have cancer as a preexisting condition. If you're already in treatment, ask your health care provider's office staff to suggest some options. If you're not, you may qualify for Medicaid or (in New York State) Family Health Plus. The social services department of your local hospital will have applications for these programs.

HELP FROM UNCLE SAM

The 1996 Health Insurance Portability and Accountability Act (HIPAA) protects you when you want to switch, keep, or buy new health insurance. HIPAA limits exclusions on preexisting conditions in group health plans; gives new enrollees credit for prior coverage; makes it illegal to use health status as a reason for denying health coverage; guarantees group coverage for employers with fifty or fewer employees; and guarantees renewability of group health plans. For more on HIPAA's provisions, have a look at www.health insuranceinfo.net.

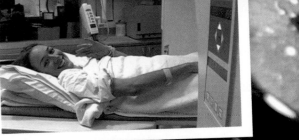

IT'S SCAN DAY:
time to kick cancer's ass!

Now that the insurance tour is over, it's time to load up the tools you've picked up in Cancer College and get ready to meet your treatment challenges head-on.

First among them has got to be the anxiety that leads up to scan day. You sweat blood!

On the day itself, expect the stress volume to be turned up to full blast and your internal woofers to blow out. Here's some advice that will hopefully help you turn it down a notch or two.

tip no.26

SCHEDULE YOUR SCANS EARLY IN THE MORNING
so you don't have to fast all day

If you're like me, you hate to miss a meal. You may have to make your appointments several months in advance, so don't forget this one. Another reason why it's worth it to get up early: If you press, you may be able to get your results the same day and thwart the overnight panic. But tread lightly, and have manners. Remember Nurse Ratchet? Well, dealing with pushy, holier-than-thou wenches probably didn't make her attitude any better.

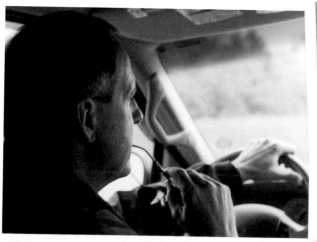

Doppler Dad, my navigator

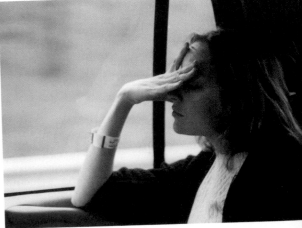

Scan day stress

tip no.27

BRING TONS OF TRASHY FLUFFY MAGAZINES
to help you escape...

If possible, contact your doctor's office to find out if he or she is running late. Waiting rooms can be pretty depressing, so you want to limit your time there as much as possible. But if you're stuck, lose yourself in nonsense. It's too hard to focus on smart stuff, so give yourself a break. Follow Brad and Angelina's latest global kid-shopping spree or Britney's party-animal lush fests. Don't rely on the hospital to be au courant with its entertainment rags. If you do, you'll most likely be stuck with battered issues of *Redbook* and *Ladies' Home Journal* from the late 1990s. Or worse, *Golf!* That's just torture.

tip no.28

WEAR A SPORTS BRA
with no metal in it

This way you can avoid flashing boob every time you lift an arm or adjust your position on the CAT scan bed. I swear hospital gowns were designed by a man! No matter how stylish you are with your Jimmy Choo heels, top-shelf jeans, and I'm-a-survivor lipstick with names like "Courageous Spirit" and "Strength," the second you don the gown you feel sick, exposed, and utterly style-less. Some hospitals have upgraded to robes and trousers, but others still rely on the bare-backed, easy-exit—or, God forbid, entry—design. Where did they get those patterns, kindergarten art class? If you find yourself in this shame-inducing predicament, ask for a second robe to cover your derriere. Otherwise you'll leave no mystery behind (so to speak) as you sashay from vitals to radiology.

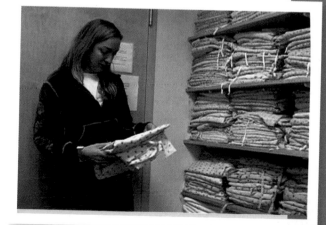

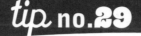

tip no.29

BRING ALONG A
cancer pal

CHEMO ANGELS

During chemo you need as many angels hovering over you as possible. If you'd like to add to your angel posse, check out this Web site: www.chemo angels.net. This group matches patients who are going through the difficult time of chemo with angels who, through little notes, cards, and small gifts, seek to deliver a bit of cheer and encouragement.

Ask a friend or a relative to accompany you to your doctor's appointments. In my case it's a great time for a family reunion—sans the picture albums and gin-and-tonics! Ask your cancer pal to take notes for you (or, if you just can't find somebody to go with you, bring a tape recorder). This way you won't be stuck being the cancer courtroom stenographer. You may only have a few minutes with your doctor. If you get overwhelmed, you'll probably miss some important information. Backup ears (and a compassionate shoulder in case the tears flow) are a must!

tip no.30

SCHMOOZE WITH THE
hospital staff

Befriend the phlebotomist. She's the gal (for some reason it's never a dude) who sticks you for a blood draw. If you're sweet, she may think twice before taking her recent divorce out on your arm. Also be chipper with the vitals gal—the one who takes your blood pressure and temperature and records the dreaded weigh-in. With a little convincing she may let you shave off those last ten pounds of shoe and lipstick weight.

HOSPITAL HOSPITALITY

Keep a bowl of candy—primo stuff—in your room for your guests and nurses. You'll be surprised just how many drive-bys you'll get at just the moment when the remote slips or the ice is empty.

tip no.31

BEFRIEND A *stewardess*

Thanks to chemo you may have to add "vomit bag" to your list of cancer accessories. If you're not able to charm a stewardess into loading you up, here are some resources for emergency chemo-induced projectiles:

- **Chick Sick Sacks at www.chemo chicks.com run $10–20. "Don't let a little queasiness keep you at home," the site says. "When the nausea gets tough, the tough get Sick Sacks!"**

- **If you're not looking to spend a lot, for a measly fifty cents you can purchase a Sic-Sac Motion Sickness Bag at www.flightessentials.net.**

- **For a sporty, discreet, upscale barf bag, go to www.redebag.com.**

- **Good ol' Walgreens offers a stash of "convenience bags" on its site at www.walgreens.com.**

- **If you're looking for a bag with a little British flair, take a gander at the English Web site www.chuckiebags.com.**

- **And lastly, if it's a reliable, no-frills barf bag you're searching for, look no farther than www.sicksaver.com. However, with a puking stick figure on the outside, they may draw a little more attention than you'd like.**

tip no.32

TAKE THE FIFTY CENT *tour*

Besides being a mega-talented photographer and fancy editor at *Glamour* magazine, Suzanne Donaldson is also my wonderful cousin. Less than four months after she married her terrific husband, Steve, she was diagnosed with hairy cell leukemia, a rare blood cancer that literally produces hairy-looking cells, which lunch on the healthy ones. I guess we can officially say cancer with crazy names runs in our family now. Great, crack the champagne.

Suzanne offers some great advice on how to prepare yourself for your first day of treatment: Ask beforehand to see the chemo room and any other location where you will be spending time, so you know what to expect. It can be a shocker if you don't.

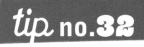

Suzanne:
I wish, I wish, I wish they had just walked me down the hall on a calm day to check the place out before I started

61

PROFILE:
SUZANNE DONALDSON

suzanne's icon:

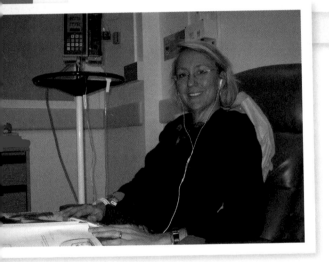

AGE: 45

HAIR COLOR: Blond!

EYES: Blue

HEIGHT: 5'9"

WEIGHT: 126 after colonic

HOMETOWN: Originally Washington, D.C., but now New York City

OCCUPATION: Photo director, *Glamour* magazine

FAVORITE SAYING: "Let it go."

BEST TIP: Pick an icon or some kind of touchstone to remind you of your aspirations every day. For me, it's the Statue of Liberty. She is my metaphor for a strong, powerful woman.

treatment. I know I would have been better prepared if I'd had a mental image of where they were taking me and what was about to happen. But no. Instead, my first day was a super-long one filled with EKGs and countless check-ins.

I remember being in a waiting room filled with patients of all ages and with varying degrees of cancer. Not a fun place to be. We sat in the corner watching all these sick people and their spouses or partners with them. It didn't seem that we belonged there. When I was finally called to go into the chemo room, it hit me. My month of cancer—which until now seemed like a distant topic that didn't belong to me, something I was just being informed about—suddenly became very real. Freak-out time! The tears welled up and then flowed out with hysterical punctuations. I felt like screaming, "Get me out of here! I do not feel sick! I don't need this, stop looking at me with such sad faces! I'm terrified and I don't want to do this!"

When they brought us into the chemo room, I officially lost it! Tears came streaming out with little air in between my sobs. This was it; I was now going to have to go through with fixing it. "It" being this thing inside me that I couldn't even feel and hardly seemed real.

What I'll describe next was scary, mainly because I wasn't prepared. The staff directed me to the chemo chair. An IV shunt was then put into the top of my arm, where they also did a blood test. Then they started me off with a little saline to flush my veins, followed by a custom cocktail; in my case it was cladribine that dripped through my veins for several hours. My tears continued to flow. My husband freaked out and then crashed. All this was followed by a peanut butter and jelly sandwich on white bread, lots of water, and a mountain of trying hard to forget my troubles.

more chemo tips FROM SUZANNE

- Bring a good pal or family member to your chemo treatments (one you actually like spending time with).

- Take an iPod or portable CD player to drown out all the sounds around you.

- Bring a blanket or throw of some kind—these rooms can get very chilly.

- Pack lots of water and a healthy snack—fruit, nuts, baby carrot sticks.

- Rest! Chemo takes it out of you (quite literally), so take it easy and lick your wounds.

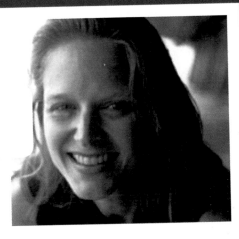

heidi's icon:

PROFILE:
HEIDI ADAMS

AGE: 39 (pushing young adulthood as far as I can)

HAIR COLOR: Blond

EYES: Blue

HEIGHT: 5'8"

WEIGHT: Information released on a need-to-know basis (meaning only to doctors who are prescribing meds or to the treadmill at the gym)

HOMETOWN: Austin, Texas

OCCUPATION: Founder/executive director of Planet Cancer; mother of twins

FAVORITE SAYING: "Don't forget to breathe."

BEST TIP: Be absolutely present in every moment. If you're working, work. If you're with your kids or husband, really be with them instead of being distracted by a million other things. And never miss a chance to say "thank you," "well done," or "I love you."

DON'T GET STEAMROLLERED BY THE
hospital routine

The coolest thing about cancer (yes, there are silver linings) is the people you meet who may never have come into your life without the bridge of this disease. My honorary twin Heidi Adams is one of those people. We're not actually related, but everyone thinks we were separated at birth because we share a similar dose of naughty and nice. She's the only person I will share my secret perfume combo potion with. Heidi founded Planet Cancer—a community for young adults (defined in the cancer world as anyone from fifteen to forty years old) with cancer. As she puts it, it's for that age between "pediatric" and "geriatric," where no one knows whether to give you a lollipop or have a serious talk about your fiber intake! When Heidi was twenty-six she was diagnosed with Ewing's sarcoma, a rare bone cancer that typically occurs in children. Here are some choice nuggets from her treatment experiences.

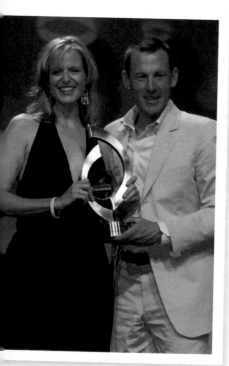

With Lance Armstrong

Heidi:

When packing for my stays in the center where I received my treatments every six weeks or so, I included tons of magazines because I didn't have the attention span for books. When I checked in, the first thing I did was put a sign on the door: NO PAPER. NO TRAYS. NO ICE. I WEIGH 135 POUNDS. This was to keep people from waking me up at the crack of dawn. I found it important to ferret out what was important and what was just stupid hospital bureaucratic routine, and to refuse any invasiveness that wasn't absolutely necessary. For fun, I used to crank-call the nurses, especially after one experience: I had started to feel pretty achy and feverish. The night nurse came in and I said, "I feel achy and feverish." She said, "Have you been around any sick people lately?" I just looked at her and started howling with laughter, as I gasped, "You mean besides all these cancer patients?!"

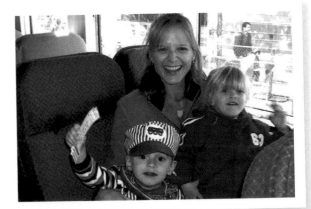

Heidi and her twins

HEIDI: PLANET CANCER

I started Planet Cancer because I didn't think that other young women and men should experience the same kind of isolation I felt when I went through treatment. I met only four people my own age during my entire fourteen months of treatment—only through random chance, not through any of the formal support mechanisms. Even worse, three of them died. I was surrounded by people my grandparents' age. Not that they weren't very nice people going through their own difficulties, but they just couldn't relate to the problems I faced at my stage of life. Things like not dating, feeling like my friends' lives were moving forward and mine was on hold, facing mortality for the first time, moving back in with my parents and depending on them again, facing the potential loss of my fertility.

After I started Planet Cancer in 2000 and got further into it, I realized that younger adults were falling through the cracks on a whole different level: We are the least represented group in clinical trials, we're more likely to experience a delayed diagnosis, and our overall survival rates have not improved in thirty years. So in addition to providing mechanisms for peer support, Planet Cancer advocates for younger adults with cancer and, hopefully, empowers our members to advocate for themselves individually. For more details, go to www.planetcancer.org.

tip no.34

MOVING IN??
well then, renovate!

So if you have to stay in the hospital or other treatment facility for longer than just a slumber party, move in! You'll feel much more comfortable if you're surrounded by your stuff. Why not decorate? I'm always happier when my nest is cozy. If your temporary home is an antiseptic box, then turn it into a glam palace, English garden, or Swiss chalet. Perhaps you'd prefer to be in Bali or Singapore? Wherever it is you'd rather be, create it! Bring your own pillow and comforter, some slippers, and a soft robe. Surround yourself with pictures of the people you love and the things that inspire you. Vibe is everything, so grab some Christmas lights and create the mood for healing.

COLLECT (OR MAKE)
designer gowns

As we've already discussed, hospital chic is an oxymoron. But why wear the regulation hospital blue or gray when you can create a smashing Diane von Furstenberg "hostess gown" knockoff? Time for a little sewing task, Project Runway style! Invite your Cancer Posse to participate and make it a girlie craft night. You can download patterns off the Internet at www.lazygirldesigns.com or modify an existing dress of your own. Go ahead, get out the needle, thread, and glue guns, ladies! Just remember—no metals. Unfortunately brass, steel, silver, or sterling sequins can't go through the scan machine (it's magnetic). But your in-room gown can—and should—be bedazzling! Here are some items you can use to embellish your gown for a totally unique look:

- **Ribbons** (upgrade the scraggly ties with bold flare)
- **Buttons,** vintage and new (think Chanel)
- **Vintage fabric** cut into cute shapes (Bohemian chic)
- **Small mirrors** (Bollywood chic)
- **Suede or leather fringe** (Montana chic)
- **Flower appliqués** (just don't overdo it. Laura Ashley went out in the 1980s.)
- **Beaded trim** (elegant and simple)

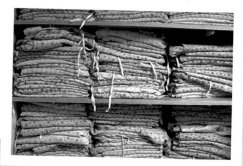

HEALING THREADS

If you're not feeling particularly crafty but you still want a stylish gown to wear to the hospital ball, check out this Web site: www.spirited-sisters.com. The dignified collection of gowns available on this site comes in a spectrum of colors, including purple, pink, and green. Plus, you can choose from a variety of styles like "the casual," the elegant," or "the wrap." The gowns are a fabulous alternative to the indignity of standard hospital garb. Detailing includes interior front pockets that act as "a safe and secure haven for personal items or drainage bags," and slash pockets that allow wearers "to tuck away personal items, or to give themselves a hug!" The gowns come complete with soft back closures that allow "access to just enough."

remember:

Understand the basics of exactly what cancer is and isn't.

Nobody can predict the future. Don't be gunned down by what you hear. Incurable isn't a declaration, it's a dare.

Approach your cancer fight as if it were your very own business start-up. The mission statement of your new company: Kick ass!

Round up the best team of doctors and healers possible.

Travel outside your town or city, your state, or even the country to find the best treatment possible.

Not every doctor you visit is going to be a perfect match. Shop around and don't settle for less than the best.

Seek second and third opinions!

Assign tasks to family and friends to help lighten your load and keep you organized.

Create and maintain a medical binder to keep information and medical documents orderly.

Understand your insurance coverage and insurance options.

Schedule your scans in the morning so you don't have to fast all day. Bring trashy magazines along to help you escape.

Ask a friend or relative to accompany you to your doctor's appointments. If you must go alone, bring a tape recorder.

Before going for treatment, take a tour of the treatment facility so you'll know what to expect.

If you have to sign up for an extended stay in a hospital or treatment facility, decorate! Surround yourself with things you love and that make you comfy.

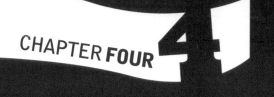

when do I become
A SURVIVOR?

{ survivor isn't just a term — it's an attitude }

Survivors are like tea bags: You don't know how strong we are until you dip us in hot water. So when do you get to call yourself a survivor? Today, mamacita, today! A survivor is a person who perseveres despite hardship or danger. Isn't that you? This may seem like a chapter that should come toward the end of the book, but for many folks living with cancer is a day-to-day, ongoing challenge. Each of you has the right to define your own journey. Go with what feels right for you.

**In my mind, you are a survivor
the day you are diagnosed.**

So don't be timid, say it loud and say it proud. There's no need to wait for the green light from Mr. Doctor Man. Celebrate! Crack the bubbly and order a three-tiered organic frosted cake. Make sure it's fattening and share it with no one. Go ahead, I dare you, walk over to the mirror and say it! I am a survivor.

REPLACE THE WORD *PATIENT* WITH
the word survivor

I didn't always feel this way. In fact, up until recently I didn't dare use the S-word. That was a special term reserved for remarkable, strong people. "Survivors" belonged to a ritzy, dress-code-only country club, a place where the jet-setting cancer-free toasted themselves and hobnobbed. "Dahhhhling, I'm a survivor, pass the Grey Poupon." I wanted so badly to join. But there I was, nose pressed against the window, envious. In my mind the only way through the emerald gates was remission, or perhaps a job as a dishwasher or caddy. Why not? Didn't the elite survivor set need someone to haul their burdens once they laid 'em down? I'd gladly schlep stuff for the opportunity to be on the other side of sick.

As women with cancer we live every day with an indescribable weight on our shoulders.

We tiptoe on the razor-edge of mortality, one hand touching the heavens, the other grabbing the earth. We juggle dying with living while paying the bills, doing the grocery shopping, picking up the kids, changing the oil, fixing that damn leaky pipe that warped the new floors, and coping with the boss from hell to whom we refuse to reveal any signs of cancer weakness. Are we not "surviving" while managing the demands of a busy life? The planet doesn't stop and wait for us to get well, so why should we? And why should anyone define us as anything other than the dynamic hot tomatoes that we are?

Whether you've made it through the battle or are still in the trenches, pink hats, special ribbons, and raised hands for everyone—not just the "winners." When I started to call myself a survivor, my whole attitude changed. I put cancer behind me (even though it was still full-blown Stage IV) and started living again.

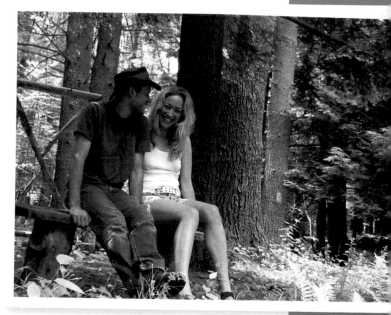

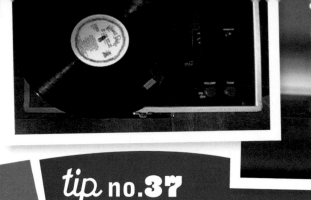

tip no.37

PLAY GLORIA GAYNOR'S "I WILL SURVIVE" SO LOUD
that the neighbors call the cops

I love to dance barefoot, play air guitar in my underpants, and sing (badly) in the shower. It makes me feel free. Sometimes I pretend I'm a Vegas showgirl dripping with sequins and gold lamé. I imagine that the more embarrassed and foolish I feel, the greater the healing power. Daily shower concerts echo through my house. (Note: Hairbrushes make great microphones.) My shows make me high on life. Maybe I should forget about this writing thing and go on the road! I mean, who else can cluck out Led Zeppelin's "Whole Lotta Love" with such passion and heart? You're never too sick to air-guitar! Even if you're bed-bound, move those toes to the rhythm, sing along with your iPod or boom box, and—as they say in the beginning of the Martin Scorsese flick *The Last Waltz*—play it loud!

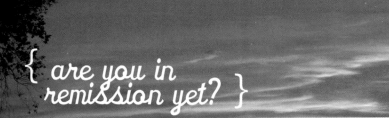

{ are you in remission yet? }

That term remission can be confusing. We all want to use it. We beg and make promises to the higher-ups for the privilege to include it in our self-describing vocabulary. But some-times it just doesn't apply—or it isn't the winner-take-all lottery we imagined it to be, especially since cancer treatments can often leave us with neurological disorders, chronic fatigue, sexual impairment, premature meno-pause, low self-esteem, and the traumatizing anxiety of a relapse. Sheesh! Are the mighty women who will never be in remission lost in the purgatory of the permanent patient? Or worse, the victim? That's a big no-no.

One of the first questions people asked when they found out I was writing a book and making a film about my cancer journey was "Did you beat cancer? Are you in remis-sion yet?" Yet? Oh, the pressure! At first that dreaded question took the wind out of my sails.

It felt invasive and nosy, as if I were being quizzed on my net worth or, worse, my weight! But on a deeper level, I was just ashamed to admit that I hadn't kicked it yet. If I had only tried harder, maybe I'd be in the popular clique. Truth be told, I just hated making people worry and light candles. I wanted it all behind me.

tip no.38

CREATE YOUR OWN *cancer term*

REMISSION: *no signs of cancer left in your body.*

CURED: *after five years of remission, you are considered cured.*

If neither of these terms apply to you, don't fret—create your own! I used to bang my head against the wall trying to come up with ways to explain the cancer I have to people.

As hard as I tried, I was never successful. They'd scratch their heads and give me that confused what's-gonna-happen-to-you look. But as soon as I invented the term *progression-free remission*—lazy and (thankfully) unproductive tumors that just hang out like couch potatoes—they got it. Deep sigh! I ran it by Dr. D, and he thought it was both creative and spot-on. So I'm starting a club of my own, and if you've got a cancer like the one I have, you're invited to join. We laugh too loud, accessorize with glitter, and believe deeply in the power of honky-tonk.

Admittedly, I felt a little funny using my new term at first—like I was a phony, masquerading as someone that I wasn't. Then I thought: What if I jinxed myself? Was I just asking for trouble? Or what if I did become cancer-free one day; would years of using my term make it anticlimactic? Like saying you're sixteen when you're really fifteen and a half or opening all your presents on Christmas Eve? I mean, once the carnage is over you fall into a big depression because you know all that's left for the merry morning is a stocking full of toothbrushes, antibacterial soap, and hand warmers. Hooray.

After a while I realized that my term *progression-free remission* was a necessary coping tool for a chronic disease that I might have to manage for the rest of my life. Hey, whatever works!

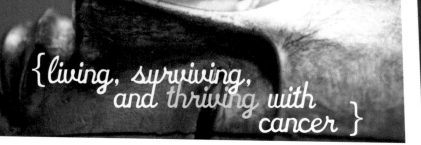

Though it might not seem like it, this is the time to start taking some risks and planning for your future. That's right, your future isn't a luxury. There are no crystal balls, and magic carpets are just too hard to clean, so stop wasting time and start having fun! Cancer or not, we all know what it's like to long for something. Most of us spend the better part of our twenties and thirties longing for Mr. or Ms. Right and the perfect job. Once we nab

that, it's off to pining for that dream house (or apartment for you urban dwellers out there). How many times do we think of our lives as *really* starting when "this" happens?

Why does it take a challenge to our survival for us to give ourselves permission to really live?

Why don't we accept the gift of life as our birthright?

tip no.39

MAKE A LIST OF 10 THINGS YOU'VE ALWAYS WANTED TO DO *and try them*

I call this exercise "New Year's Resolutions in June." Write down the first thing that comes to mind and post it someplace where you can see it. Don't get stuck in practicalities, and don't edit. Painting? Cooking? Writing? Skydiving? Karate? Learning a new language? Your only limitation is your imagination. I like to take flaming red lipstick and write mine on mirrors. Each time I obsessively scrutinize myself (as my dad used to say, "You're still there!"), I am reminded to make peace with my cellulite and focus on what's important, what my resolutions represent: living the life I want.

This exercise may seem silly, like a hokey self-help waste of time. But it's a bridge from you to your inner kid, the neglected little scruff who really needs to play because cancer grown-ups are just way too serious! In fact, when you feel a tantrum coming on, it's probably your restless inner kid reminding you to lighten up. Be juicy and courageous, take off the shackles, and set some goals. If you want to up the ante, give yourself a time line. Dream big, but save room and be flexible. Your ultimate plan may be even better than the one you can imagine! And remember the old saying, "Be careful what you wish for."

Okay, so the cancer-free part didn't stick to my plan, and I didn't go to Cuba or Vietnam, but it's spooky how many of the other things happened, like selling my film, writing this book, and meeting and marrying a righteous dude! Guess the powers that be thought *Damn, this chick has big demands. But what the heck, she's been through a lot; let's grant her a few wishes.*

Trade in the excuses for why-the-hell-nots!

We can change the trajectory of our lives no matter what seemingly insurmountable obstacles stand in our way. Here's the key: Abandon the nagging stinkin' thinkin'. You know, that silly chatter that keeps you stuck. The *I'm not this* or *I'm too that*. These thoughts are like diseases that fester. Their symptoms range from general malaise to debilitating episodes of sloth-like unworthiness. "Cancer of the noggin" I call it. It's very dangerous, but luckily there is a cure: Do what makes you feel good. If you don't like something, don't do it. And for God's sake, if you don't have something nice to say about yourself then keep your big trap shut!

> "While we have the gift of life, it seems to me that the only tragedy is to allow part of us to die—whether it is our spirit, our creativity, or our uniqueness."
>
> **—GILDA RADNER,**
> **COMEDIAN, ACTRESS**

MY FIVE-YEAR TIME LINE

When I was first diagnosed, I created a life itinerary as part of my emotional survival plan. I chose five years because that seems to be the magical cancer time frame.

2003. Move from my apartment. I've been talking about making a change forever. Do it! Plus, quit acting, shoot film, oh, and heal.

2004–2005. Cancer-free! Finish documentary. Fall madly in love with a groovy dude who has a sense of humor, is smart, creative, and loves to travel. I don't think I know him yet, but I pray he comes into my life. Maybe he's a photographer?

2006. Marry smart-ultimate-soul-mate guy. Sell film. Hit the road! What's Vietnam or Cuba like?

2007. Start working on book.

2008. Start working on family (thirty-six years old!). DOH! Can I really put all this out there? Why the heck not, it's my time line!

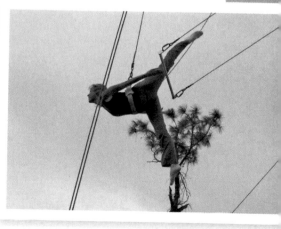

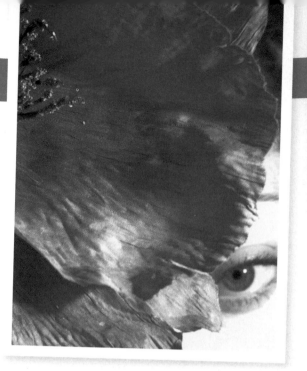

tip no.40

AWAKEN YOUR
artistic mojo!

What better way to arouse your creative mojo than with an artist date? Come on, we're girls! We love getting gussied up and hitting the town! There's just one thing: On this date you're flying solo. You don't need anybody else around distracting you or cluttering up your creative space. Even if it feels like you're squeezing blood from a stone, set aside time each week to nurture your creative side. This doesn't have to mean pulling out the paint box, camera, or journal. Pamper yourself, window-shop, watch an old movie—whatever feeds your own private muse. Think of it as playtime and defend it from all trespassing interlopers.

Each of us has an inner reservoir, a deep well from which we draw healing waters. But when we stop paying attention or extend ourselves too far, we overtap the source and drain the magic juice. If your well is depleted, then it's time to fill 'er up. Explore what interests you. Get some wine and play old records, sign up for belly-dancing classes, buy a pair of oversize sunglasses and cruise around, take a self-portrait—perhaps in the nude. (Hey, it's the age of digital, no one will see it. If you hate it, you can always hit DELETE.) Try out an exotic recipe. If you ruin it, take yourself out for dinner and laugh. Whatever you choose, make sure it fills you with the diva spirit!

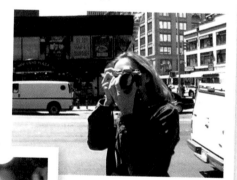

"There is a vitality, a life force, an energy, a quickening that is translated through you into action, and because there is only one of you in all time, this expression is unique. And if you block it, it will never exist through any other medium and will be lost."
— MARTHA GRAHAM, CHOREOGRAPHER

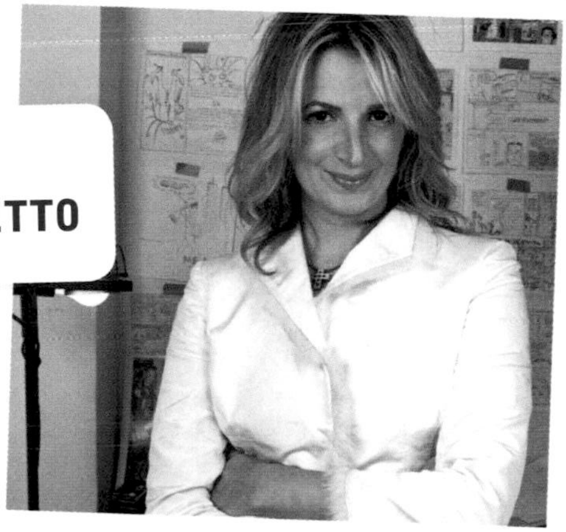

AGE: 46

HAIR COLOR: Only my colorist knows for sure

EYES: Black

HEIGHT: Tall in heels

WEIGHT: Guess

HOMETOWN: New York City

OCCUPATION: Cartoonist

FAVORITE SAYING: "Like attracts like."

BEST TIP: See the positive in everything.

marisa's icon: CANCERVIXEN

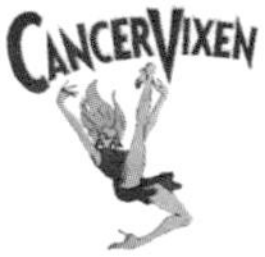

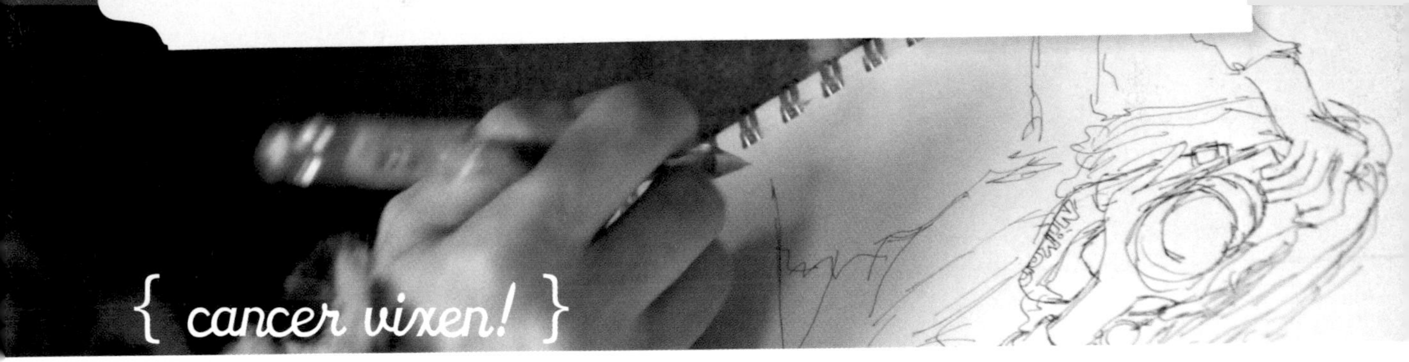

{ cancer vixen! }

Marisa:

Shortly after I was diagnosed with breast cancer, I received a call from my editor at *Glamour* magazine. I did some regular freelancing for the publication, and she was calling to check in. "What's going on in your life?" she asked. I told her about my recent diagnosis. After her initial shock, she asked me if I wanted to write about my experience for the magazine. I immediately realized that's exactly what I wanted to do. It just made perfect sense. Everything I do is autobiographical in a way anyway, and truth be told, I had already started taking notes. The cartoon spread I ultimately did for *Glamour* morphed into a graphic memoir published by Alfred A. Knopf.

At first I didn't know what title to give my story. My initial title was "Breast

Case Scenario." But thanks to a close friend of mine, that was nixed. We were having coffee and I ran "Breast Case Scenario" past him. Without pulling any punches he said it was horrible. In fact, he looked me up and down and said, "Look at you! Look what you're wearing! You look like a victim! You're walking around in sweatpants and sneakers. Go home and put on your shoes, be a Vixen! In fact, that's what you should call your book: *Cancer Vixen!*" And so *Cancer Vixen* was born.

Working on the story while I was going through treatment for my cancer made the whole experience less intimidating. *Cancer Vixen* tells the story of my eleven-month battle with cancer. The book was billed as "What happens when a shoe-crazy, lipstick-obsessed, wine-swilling, pasta-slurping fashion fanatic with a fabulous life finds a lump in her breast." Participating in the creative pro-

cess of putting the book together made me feel like I could and would conquer the cancer. With the book, I was able to literally laugh in the face of cancer! Like the time when my doctor was preparing to inspect my tumor and said, "We need to find out whether the cells are angry." That day I went home and drew them as little green meanies giving me the finger.

Like Marisa, my friend Oni put cancer to work as her muse. From the get-go, Oni, a successful actress, playwright, and writer, decided she would turn her experiences into art. On her list of artistic accomplishments since her diagnosis is an award-winning play she wrote about breast cancer called *Tough Titty*.

Oni:

I don't feel wise as a result of cancer, I feel more accepting of my own humanness. And in that way I feel more connected to everybody. I'm glad there is poetry, and I'm glad there's theater, because so much of this is just life and just metaphor. Everybody's got something. You either accept it, or you fight your whole life long. Now what do you want to do? Do you want to fight against what's really happening or sink into it somehow, cause there might be something valuable in there.

As an artist, my way of digesting life's events is to write. I've known for years, as events unfolded after diagnosis, that there was a useful story in each event. My play, *Tough Titty*, is wonderful. I've

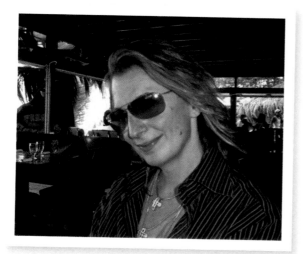

oni's icon:

PROFILE:
ONI FAIDA LAMPLEY

AGE: 40-something-ish

HAIR COLOR: Black

EYES: Brown

HEIGHT: Larger than life

WEIGHT: Not sure, I detonated my scale

HOMETOWN: Oklahoma City

OCCUPATION: Playwright and actress

FAVORITE SAYING: "You can decide you're going to learn something, but you don't get to decide what."

BEST TIP: This morning I woke up in my right mind with a reasonable portion of my good health. I feel blessed.

never said that about anything I've ever done in my life, not even a pie I've baked, but I'll say it about this play. In it a thirty-seven-year-old black woman is diagnosed with breast cancer. The play explores the toll the treatment and recurrences of the disease take on her life. In the end the character manages to give up her idea of how life is "supposed" to go.

It's been my hope that all women, but black in particular, who see the play will find a role model in the lead character. For me, when I was first diagnosed I yearned to see the faces of black women who'd survived cancer. Growing up in Oklahoma City in the '70s, I never knew anyone black who admitted she'd had it.

Surely there was someone, but people didn't talk about those things. I went to the library and saw *Celebrating Life* by Sylvia Dunnavant sticking out on the shelf. Inside were images of black survivors. Their stories filled my spiritual arsenal. I'll never ever say that I'm thankful for cancer, but the fact of the matter is that without it, I never would have written this play. Sometimes it feels like cancer is this thing that gave me this little present in a box with ribbons—the play. But now cancer has stayed too long, and I wish it would leave, just leave me the box and go away.

{ the re:writing project }

Another posse member, Jodi Sax, also embraced the therapeutic benefits of creativity. In fact, thanks to Jodi many cancer survivors were given the opportunity to chronicle their experiences for publication. Jodi is the founder of The New York LifeLab, an organization that helps cancer survivors in their twenties and thirties find mentors in the community to help them learn new skills or enter new careers. A unique writing class called the re:Writing Project is the organization's core program.

PROFILE:
JODI SAX

jodi's icon:

AGE: 39-ish and holding
(I need to be able to remain a part of my own demographic!)

HAIR COLOR: Blond

EYES: Brown

HEIGHT: 5'4"

WEIGHT: 124 (well, my chemo weight. And that's all you're going to get out of me!)

HOMETOWN: Los Angeles, California

OCCUPATION: Entertainment and intellectual property attorney; founder and executive director of LifeLab (www.nylifelab.org)

FAVORITE SAYING: "I'm doing the best I can."

BEST TIP: Pay attention to the little things in life, stand up for yourself, don't be afraid to question your doctor (and/or switch doctors if necessary).

Jodi:

I was diagnosed with colon cancer in November 2002 when I was thirty-seven. At the time I was a successful entertainment and intellectual property attorney. Initially I was told that my cancer was inoperable, and I would be given palliative care (fortunately, at the time I didn't know what palliative meant). I went on to prove the doctors wrong, and today I am cancer-free. There have been a few bumps along the way, and I certainly don't feel terrific, but I no longer have cancer.

For me, the most difficult part of the cancer experience wasn't necessarily being sick; it was living after being told I might die. I was now unable to conceive and bear children. I was too tired to get out of bed some days. And I no longer cared about clients whining about their problems. How is a person supposed to process this, especially one dealing with these issues at a time in her life when she isn't entirely settled? I found that many of my peers who had been diagnosed with cancer were looking for the same answers. So to help in the search, I started New York LifeLabs, a program designed to focus on how to live without cancer after having lived with it.

One way the organization helps members to ask and answer the life questions that arise after a diagnosis is through its re:Writing Project. The project's participants work with a professional writing instructor. Two class levels are offered. The first class teaches participants about the narrative form to give them the tools to express their voices. We teach poetry and then prose, and work on group exercises and take-home projects. A lot of the participants want to write books about their experiences, so this gives them tools. By the end we put together a long-form piece.

Also, we have mentors who volunteer to offer the students connections and help. Last year we had the editor in chief at Little, Brown, an editor from Simon & Schuster, someone from Warner Books, and an agent from William Morris. So it's pretty high-level. At the end of the class, we publish a literary journal with participants' work and have a launch party. We also have an intermediate class, which is a continuation of part one and is presented in a workshop format. It's run like a graduate school creative writing workshop (people write at home, and then their work is critiqued), with the goal of getting a piece ready for publication. And some of our participants have been published in some major places!

The goal of the class was to offer people tools to become writers, but it turned out to be a huge help emotionally to participants, and really enabled them to process some difficult stuff. People were able to write about things in ways that they were not able to talk about them. This helped to externalize the feelings and make them a bit less charged. In a way it turned the experience into art, or at least objectified it a little bit.

tip no.**41**

JOURNALING IS SELF-THERAPY
on the cheap

I love to journal; it's an inexpensive way to give myself therapy! You'd be surprised at how the simple act of transferring your thoughts onto the page allows you to tap into your inner voice. If you're new to journaling and find yourself staring down at a blank page, try a few simple exercises to break the ice and get started:

- **Using two hundred words or less,** paint a self-portrait with words.

- **What are your top five favorite things?** What are your top five least favorite things?

- **Write about someone** who has inspired you.

- **Describe** one of your happiest child-hood memories.

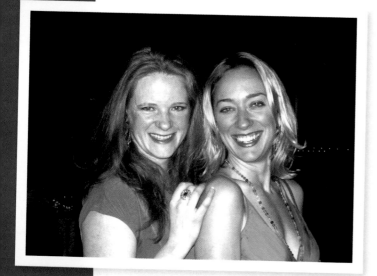

- **Write a letter to yourself** now and one from yourself ten years from now. Describe all the cool things that have happened in your life.

- **Write a letter you'll never send.**

Erin:

As a perfectionist and to-do list addict, one of the scariest things about cancer for me was the loss of control, not knowing what to expect day to day, not being able to influence the outcome of my treatment or my future. The only way I knew to gain back some of that control was to take the bad situation I was given and try to make something good come of it. For me, that meant sharing my story (in my column, at fundraisers, and eventually in my blog) and, of course, raising money and awareness for blood-related cancers, which is a whole other story. At first I just started writing everything down to get it out of my head. It was cathartic and actually removed me a bit from the situation—in some cases I felt like a reporter going deep undercover as a cancer patient. Then I realized that by simply putting myself out there, writing down my crazy, mundane, embarrassing thoughts, I was actually helping other people feel less alone. That's a great feeling. I honestly don't think I would have survived the past five years without my writing.

tip no.42

TAKE A
cancercation

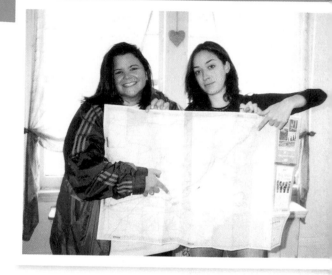

Sometimes life just whizzes by way too fast. No matter how much we get done, we're always still behind. Ever feel like your life is living you? Like the woulda-shoulda-couldas are eating you up? The constant race to relax is crazy-making. A break from your routine is what you need. When the going gets too tough . . . the tough go on vacation! Even if it's just for a long weekend, recharge your batteries on a mini soul vacation. Retreats of any kind can help you reflect and process all the changes cancer has made in your life. If you can't afford or don't feel well enough to take an extended vacation far from home, treat yourself to a more low-key getaway: a day trip antiquing or a long walk on a dusty open road. Even spending an afternoon just lying on a soft blanket in a pretty park can do wonders for the soul. What's the saying? "Sometimes you have to leave home to find it."

Before I was diagnosed, my best friend Lisa (the Google queen) and I drove from New York to Los Angeles. Lisa dreamed of writing for sitcoms while I wanted to try auditioning for pilot season on the West Coast. We stuffed nine suitcases into "Maxie," Lisa's old Nissan, and off we zoomed. It was a real Thelma-and-Louise cross-country adventure! In Virginia we lost our AAA TripTik planner (actually Lisa accidentally threw it out the window). In Tennessee we visited Graceland and were asked to leave after a botched attempt at sneaking past the ropes for a glimpse of Elvis's bedroom. We two-stepped with toothless cowboys in Arkansas, hitchhiked in Oklahoma (the car ran out of gas—oops), and strategically put our cleavage on display (well Lisa's cleavage) for a state trooper in Texas. Hey, sometimes "the girls" can get you out of a jam, especially one that involves a court date. We shared ten magnificent days sleeping in stinky motels and dining at truck stops . . . it was heaven. Then came New Mexico. The enormity of the mountains and vastness of the wide-open desert vistas made our hearts swell and our jaws drop. Two girls who could chew over every last detail of an event until all the marrow and adjectives were gone . . . were left speechless. For me it was love at first sight.

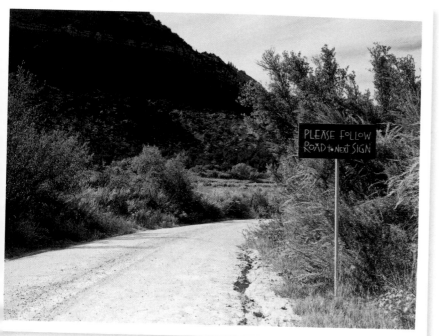

Two years after our big trip, I was diagnosed. So when it was time for my cancercation, I knew exactly where I was headed.

finding the HEALER within

I called up Lisa and asked her if she wanted to play hooky from life with me. She thought about it for all of thirty seconds and then immediately started Googling vacation rentals. Since she was between writing jobs (translation: unemployed) and I was shut down, in shock, and living off my savings, it was a perfect time to split town. We both needed to press PAUSE on our lives, and since we were finally out of debt it was a great opportunity to live off our credit cards and head west!

Our days on the road began with tea, deep conversation, and cleansing tears—"peeling the banana" we called it. I hadn't realized how much sorrow I was smushing down. I guess when your head is cluttered, it's easy to ignore the emotions that bubble just below the surface. "Inward Bound" is what we named our spiritual adventure. We went on daily pilgrimages to churches and monasteries and took in lectures and workshops. We even met a hot priest on horseback! No lie, we were hiking in the woods and out of nowhere he appeared in tight jeans and a priest collar. Wow! Maybe the church wasn't so bad after all! Lisa, a recovering Catholic, agreed.

return to ME

The trip inspired me to finally pick up my camera again. Before cancer, I had taken pictures every day. My Nikon was attached to my hip like an appendage. After my diagnosis the only image I wanted to capture was the one that held my former healthy life.

It was August, so Indian Market was in full swing in Santa Fe. Native Americans from all over the country gathered to sell their art. It was a visual feast filled with jewelry, pots, baskets, and drums. As I walked through the market, drinking in the inspiration, I felt my own creativity begin to resuscitate. Just then in the middle of the crowd, I came upon two little girls chasing each other and twirling like little dervishes, their laughter bursting through the air like tiny claps of thunder. One of the girls was Native American, the other a little blonde. They both wore braids and couldn't have been more than six or seven years old.

"My heart is jumping," one said to the other. "Is your heart jumping?"

"What?"

"Jumping!"

"Yes," I softly replied. "Yes."

As I watched them spin, I wondered what would happen if I were to spin like that. Would my heart jump so high that it shattered into thousands of tiny pieces? Maybe that's what I needed, to shatter my own heart, freeing it so that the light could shine through. Maybe everything I needed was inside me. If I could learn to quiet my mind, I could move mountains!

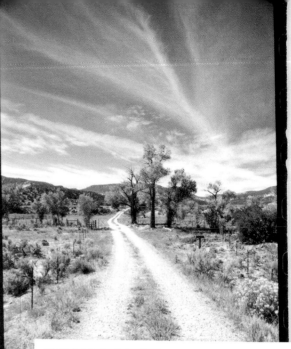

upaya and the INNER ZENDO

Nestled in the Sangre de Cristo Mountains is a beautiful Zen monastery called Upaya, a Sanskrit term that can be roughly translated as "a means." If you've ever taken a yoga class, you've experienced those annoying five minutes at the end when you're forced to inhale "let" and exhale "go." For me those last minutes were always torture. Me meditate? If I sat still, I'd snap! But when I ran across Upaya, I had a sneaking feeling that the silence within its walls would provide me the opportunity to discover what was inside me.

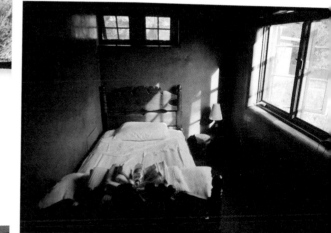

The woman who founded the monastery, Roshi Joan Halifax, had an electric way about her. I'd never seen a female monk before. She had penetrating blue eyes and a shaved head. She looked like a cool cancer survivor, only she wore robes and knew everything there was to know about the Buddha.

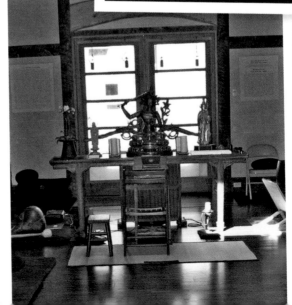

I dropped Lisa off at the airport in Albuquerque this morning and sobbed all the way back to Santa Fe. I am alone now. It's just me and I ache. Went back to the house we had just locked up, didn't know where else to go, plus I had to pee. I can't check into the Zen center until 3:00 p.m. and it's not even noon yet. I feel like an abandoned puppy in a strange place. Though I've been in Santa Fe for six weeks, nothing looks familiar. What the hell am I doing? I'm getting cold feet about my decision to volunteer for solitary Buddha confinement. Why am I so freaked out about a little meditation and alone time? It's not like I'm going to the nuthouse!

I went to a few of her meditation and dharma talks, which are conversations about how life is all an illusion and what's happening is much less important than how we relate to what's happening—get it? Though my back felt like it needed the attention of a team of chiropractors after sitting so long, I became hooked. The only problem was, it was time to leave! After six weeks, our credit cards were maxed out (again), and reality was calling. The realization I came to next sent shivers up my spine: Not only did I need to keep coming to the monastery, I needed to move in.

As I wandered aimlessly around town, killing time, I heard a faint, eerie whimper. It was a goose-bump-producing sound that seemed to be following me around. Wait, I thought, that sound is coming from me. I was letting

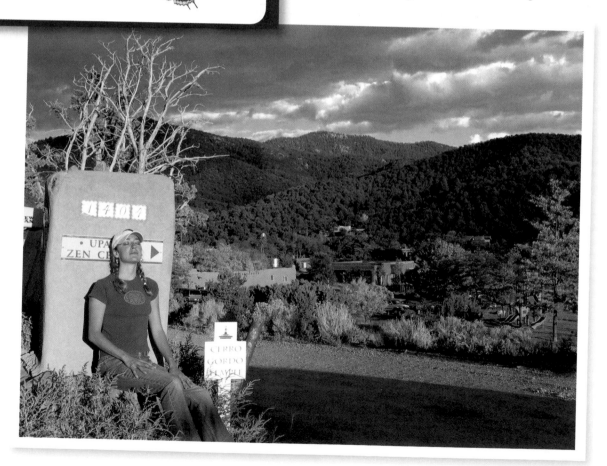

EXHALE...

Speaking of breath, ever notice how much we hold it? It's true! Most of us don't realize that we're walking around in a constant state of fight or flight. We're so accustomed to dodging bullets that we equate our high levels of stress with normalcy. Believe it or not, there is a right and a wrong way to breathe. Rapid, shallow breathing—the way most people take their oxygen in our busy society—can lead to a host of health problems, both physical and mental. Learning to breathe properly ensures that your body is getting all the yummy oxygen it needs. How do you know you're breathing right? When you're breathing properly, your stomach, not your chest, rises slightly as you breathe in. When you exhale, your stomach lowers slightly. Note: Poor posture restricts the flow of air and the rise and fall of your diaphragm. So remember your mother's nagging demands and sit up straight!

out tiny yelps of pain. Not now, please Kris, hold it together. It was 2:45, time to go! My eyes welled up as I drove up the mountain. Would I be able to say hello without bursting into tears? What would living in a Zen Buddhist monastery be like?

When I arrived, a nice woman who worked in the office showed me to my tiny (yet tasteful) spiritual cell. I dumped all my leopard luggage in the middle of the floor and wept. I cried until I was exhausted. Then I stared at the ceiling for what seemed like an eternity. Now what? Nightly meditation in the temple! Oh, what a treat. As I sat on the cushion counting my breath, the waves of emotion continued to flow. I couldn't remember the last time I'd felt so exposed. All my gunk was pouring out of me and there was no place to hide. It was embarrassing, and yet it felt good to release the weight I'd been carrying.

Après meditation, it was time for din din with the monks. Bread and soup. I was thankful for it. Until, out of nowhere, the crying started again. Stop! Stop! I begged myself to

stop but my tear ducts were on autopilot and there was no way to override the system. I dreaded the thought of being the new freak who had come to the monastery to sort out her problems, but that's exactly who I was. Thankfully the conversation at the dinner table was light. The monks had watched Margaret Cho's *Notorious C.H.O.* video and were gabbing about how it was better than *Even Cowgirls Get the Blues*. I was grateful for the un-Zen-like chatter. I had a feeling that they had seen these uncomfortable emotional episodes before and didn't want to make me feel awkward.

That night a pack of coyotes sang under my window, and I slept like a baby. The next morning everything seemed better. As the weeks went by (that's right, weeks), I blossomed. The deeper I dove, the more pearls I recovered. Beneath my junk lay a wealth of healing potential. I even learned to quiet my mind for more than four breaths! Calming my breath calmed my mind, which calmed my body. There I was, calm. Ahhh.

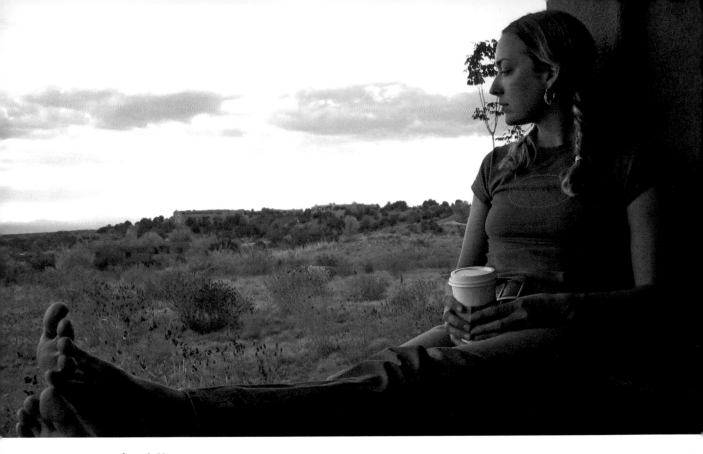

buddha CAMP

Monastery living was the opposite of the busy, hectic life I was used to. Each day at Upaya included three hour-long meditations, as well as work practices like chopping carrots, sweeping, gardening—anything that needed to be done to maintain the place. In exchange for my help and commitment, I received a room and three simple vegetarian meals (three hots and a buddha-ful cot!). Weekly intensives ranged from calligraphy to yoga and of course plenty of meditation. I loved all the classes, except one. The title alone totally gave me the creeps. It was called Being with Dying, and I vowed to make myself scarce for the roll call. Fat chance!

Just when I had learned all the correct bows and zendo etiquette (like only the head abbot gets to enter from the back of the

temple), Roshi Joan Halifax asked to see me . . . privately. *Gulp*. This was big. In fact, it had an official name, Dokasan. The protocol was very complicated. You had to bow, prostrate (three to four times, I never remembered), and chat. Then do the whole thing in reverse order and leave. Once I had finished making a fool of myself and dishonoring the tradition, I told Roshi that the Being with Dying workshop wigged me out. It made me worry that I'd manifest my death, and since I believed that worrying was praying for what you *don't* want, I didn't want to take that workshop! She laughed and promised me that it wouldn't be morbid and that if at any time I wanted to leave, I could. Translation: Get your ass to class, I'm watching you!

the "HOW TO CROAK" *workshop*

The dreaded workshop started with a writing exercise. Perfect, I thought, no meet-and-greet emotional crap! Yeah right. I wish. Within two sentences I was staining my paper with those pesky eyeball water droplets.

1. **What's the best-case scenario** for your death? (That I don't die!)

2. **What's the worst-case scenario** for your death? (Oh, give me a break!)

3. **How do your body and mind feel** after this exercise? (How do you think? Shitty!)

4. **How do you want to die** and who will be there? (I don't want to die; I want to get out of this stupid workshop!)

5. **What do you have to let go of** so that the best-case scenario can happen?

Okay, I got it: This workshop wasn't about dying, it was about exploring all the emotional sandpaper that was making living so raw and scratchy. So I stayed.

BECOME A PYROMANIAC

The night of the workshop I lit a little bonfire in the woods and burned that writing exercise. As I watched the paper roll up and disintegrate, I imagined my worries (and my tumors) melting like little ice balls. It was a good visual, especially the part about the tumors. Writing your fears on paper and reducing them to ash is a surprisingly satisfying way to release them to the universe.

tip no.43

TAKE SOME TIME TO *quiet your mind*

I was shocked at what little control I had over my mind. It was constantly traveling in a gazillion directions. I could count my breaths, order shoes online, make promises to stop avoiding the gym, and think about the foxy meditator guy three cushions to my right. Does he have a girlfriend? Is he gay? I bet he does this all the time; I really have to do this all the time. . . . If thinking was a form of talking, boy was I a chatterbox! Here are some strategies for learning to quiet the inner chitchat:

- **Concentrate on clearing your mind.** Think of your head like a champagne glass: If it's filled to the rim with nonsense, then there's no room for the joie de vivre.

- **Find a comfortable seat** (a pillow, a chair, even your bed) and scan your body for any tension. Make adjustments as necessary.

- **Now stay put and focus on one point.** You can count your breaths, stare at a candle, or listen to music. If you're using your breath, the inhale and exhale are considered one count. Try to get to ten counts without breaking into a

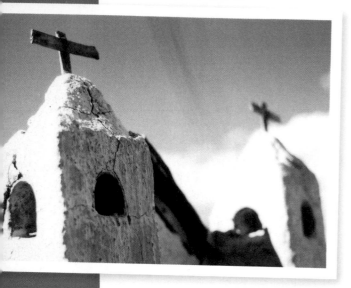

mental circus. If your mind wanders, bring it back and start over again.

- **Use a timer** so that you're not constantly wondering if you should look at your watch to see if your five minutes are up.

- **The more you work to quiet your mind, the better you'll get.** If you dabble in it like a hobby, you'll get hobby results. Like all the other parts of your body that you don't want to let sag, your mind needs regular exercise!

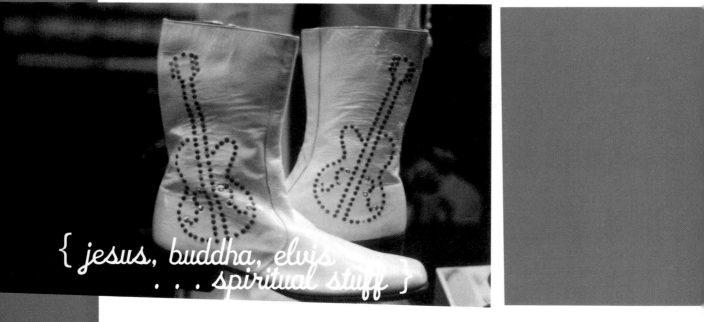

{ jesus, buddha, elvis . . . spiritual stuff }

Prayer is another way to fill your well, and the best way to pray is whatever way works for you. But just because you're sick doesn't mean you need to find your savior. If prayer helps, start chatting. If it doesn't, big whoop, make no judgments. Spirituality is a very personal trip.

In my mind there is only one temple, one church, one mosque. We each go there in our own special way. It's an inner sanctum where you and your God high-five and catch up like old buds. Traditional religions don't resonate with everyone. There's this preconceived notion that when you are diagnosed, a lightbulb goes off and you suddenly realize what it's all about. You enjoy "the moment" more and live each day like it's your last. Easier said than done. I still scream at cabs and pout when my

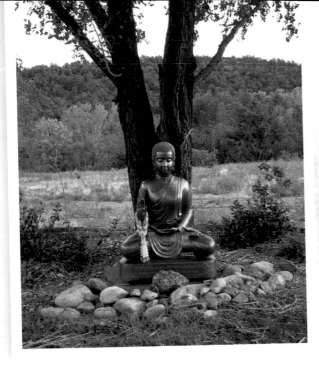

"By letting go it all gets done."
—LAO-TZU, TAOIST SAGE

husband won't share the remote. I freak out when I gain a pound and constantly wish that I didn't have such a "distinguished" profile.

There was a saying during World War I: "There are no atheists in foxholes." At first I figured there wouldn't be any in cancer wards, either. I tried to get really spiritual. I figured I was dying so I'd better hurry up and get my act together! I even purchased a few flowy frocks. Why not look the part? Maybe my new wardrobe would help with my holy transformation. "Sure she has cancer, but what a wise sage she's become. I bet she knows something I don't." Not quite. I wore my pseudo-spiritual outfits twice, but since they made me feel like a middle-aged lesbian hippie, it was back to the ripped jeans and cowboy boots, simple but elegant.

I grew up part Christian and part Wizard. God was confusing. One minute we were lighting candles and saying the rosary, and the next we were writing down names of annoying people and putting them in the freezer.

Let's just say, you didn't want to get on my Abuelita's bad side—she'd ice you out! When I was in second grade, she taught me about tarot cards and hexes. I remember trying to practice on the mean girls at the playground, but my spells must have backfired because everyone got boobs but me!

On obligatory holidays I was attacked with a comb and forced to wear a dress for church. For a tomboy like me, this was disastrous. I can still feel my (then) bony butt aching from the splintery wooden bench. Church equaled boredom. Luckily my grandma felt the same way, so the torture only took place biannually. The day I turned seven, my mother announced that I could pick my own religion. "Great!" I said. "I want to be Jewish." She froze. I had no idea what being Jewish meant; I just knew that presents and a big party were involved. Carving out my religious territory seemed like a big waste of time. In my mind I was God, a belief I shared with my sister when she turned five. It was great (and handy)! I had my very own personal congregation (aka slave) until my parents caught on and told me to "Cut it out!"

Lots of people pound their fists and yell at God. I never wanted to, but I often wondered what it was all about. Then I started praying. Now, I hesitate to use that word, because for me it was more like talking to my peeps on the other side. Sometimes they even talked back! No joke. After Grandma died, I asked her for some important heavenly advice, and I swear she said, "Eat more beans." What do you expect from a Colombian?

That's what works for me. What speaks to you? What makes you flow? What gives you comfort? You can find Jesus, Buddha, Elvis, or whoever, anywhere. Custom-design your spiritual trip. Remember, you alone have to do this work, but you don't have to do it alone. The trees can be your church. You can even find a spiritual practice in your relationships. A beach chair can be your holy ground or a cafe your ashram. It doesn't matter. The divine spirit is a wild pinto kicking inside you. Let her run.

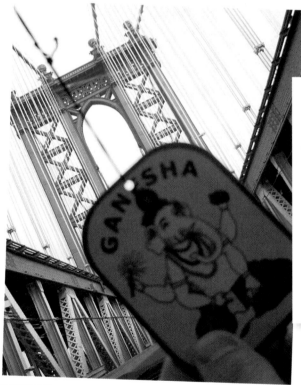

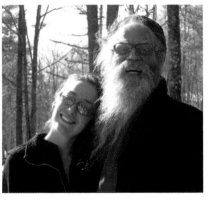

"It always comes back to just letting go with love. Just put the love in it. Whatever it is, and if you can't put love in it, don't do it!"

—BHAGAVAN DAS, SPIRITUAL GURU

tip no.44

DO WHAT MAKES YOU FEEL BETTER
and gives you hope

Marisa:

My experience battling cancer reawakened my spiritual side. Before, I felt like all that spiritual stuff didn't matter; now I realize that everything matters. What you put out into the universe is what you get back. For one thing, cancer brought me back to being Catholic. When I was going through treatment, I had all of my friends and a church praying for me. But what really worked for me, and what still works for me, is kabbalah. I am in love with kabbalah. I go quietly to the center in the middle of the day and I have my one-on-one with my rabbi. Sometimes I go to classes, but usually I just do my own thing. That's how I nourish my spiritual side, but my advice to other women battling cancer is to do what makes you feel better and gives you hope. If it feels like crap, then don't do it. Don't do it because you feel like you should do it, do it because you want to do it!

Oni:

More than ten years after my initial diagnosis, I feel more grounded in a version of the faith I had as a child—that basically it's a benign, benevolent universe. I have always believed and I still believe that I was not brought here to suffer. So if I'm only caught up in the cancer diagnosis, which involves suffering, then I'll be missing something. I believe there has to be more to it. But now after nearly a decade on this cancer trip, I know it's not my job to try and force the good juice out of it. I know that I can decide if I'm going to learn something, but I can't decide what that something is.

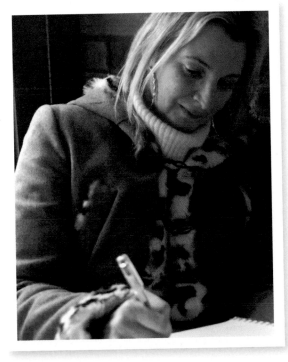

tip no.45

TAKE A MOMENT AND ACKNOWLEDGE THE CO-SURVIVORS
in your life

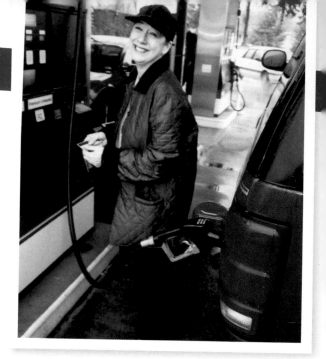

Co-survivors are the Crazy Sexy Cancer Angels, the wonderful family, best friends, and even pets who stick by your side and care for you through thick and thin. They are the sturdy behind-the-scenes folks who make the show go on. These people have grit, grace, and backbone. Let them know how thankful you are—they need to hear it. Often a simple gesture, a heartfelt note, or a special little gift will show your appreciation.

Just as we think that no one can understand what we go through, the same holds true for the people who sit in the fire with us. Often they are challenged not only emotionally, but also physically, spiritually, and financially. Before I sold my apartment to help pay for my alternative treatments, my parents shelled out the big cash in search of a cure. My mother stood right by my side. She knew how isolated

I felt, and she didn't want me to go on my hunt alone. We drove all over the country searching for answers.

We enrolled in crazy courses, fasted, tuned our chakras, beat Indian drums, and clanged Tibetan bowls. We left no stone unturned. My mom even got her yoga certification, which shocked us all. This is a woman who never broke a sweat; instead she "glowed." This is also a woman who doesn't do anything half-

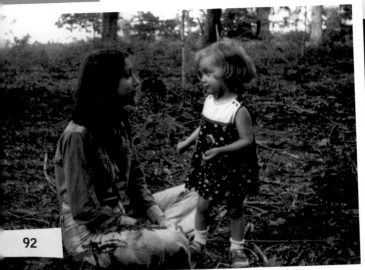

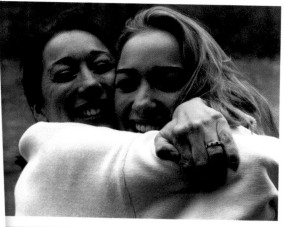

assed. So at fifty-three she became a professional yogini. My diagnosis had catapulted her into alternative living (and overachieving) panic mode.

One healer we visited charged us $800 for a two-hour meeting. He gave me a few remedies and told me I'd be cured in six months. Wow, six months! How come the rest of the world didn't know about this? He had autographs from famous celebrities like John Lennon and Gwyneth Paltrow on the wall. I was hooked. With thousand-watt smiles we thanked him profusely and headed toward the door. That's when we noticed the two packs of Marlboro reds sitting on his altar next to pictures of his wife and daughter (both of whom died of cancer). Way to take the wind out of our sails!

In my four years of living with cancer, I've only seen my mom break once. On this particular day I was reminded that she was more than just my healing sidekick, she was my parent, and her job above all else was to be protective.

"Sweet Pea"—that's what she calls me—"I'm worried that you're becoming too rigid with your alternative treatments. I see you putting yourself in a prison, and I want to help mastermind a jailhouse break."

"Mom, trust me. Please support me and don't second-guess what I try. You know there's no cure for my condition and that all I can do is my very best."

"You're right, I'm sorry, I just want you to be happy."

Later that day she came to me teary-eyed. "It's not that I don't trust your judgment, it's just that, at what point is all this healing sucking the life out of you? We need a break."

In that moment I realized that I wasn't the only one going through this.

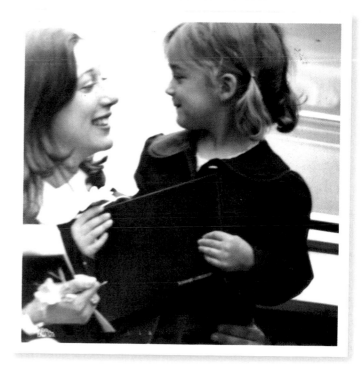

My mom and my family were survivors, too. They shared my ups as well as my downs. In their private moments, they cried, cursed, prayed, and trembled. Don't forget their feelings and pain.

Catch these important people in your life off guard; out of nowhere tell them how grateful you are. It will mean more than you know. Thank you, Mom.

> **"Courage is being scared to death, but saddling up anyway."**
> **—JOHN WAYNE, ACTOR**

tip no.46

SHOW UP FOR YOUR
co-survivors

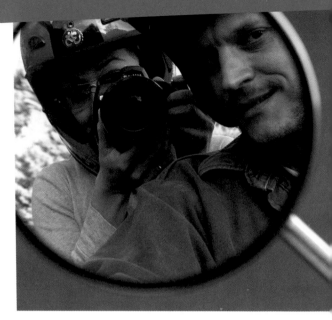

Show up, even if it's hard. Don't fall off the planet: It'll send shock waves of worry throughout your support system. Pick up the phone, send a personal e-mail, go out to dinner, check in with your relationships. Even if you don't feel like it, make time to be present for your co-survivors.

The weekend before I moved in with Brian (my then boyfriend/now righteous husband) was his twentieth high school reunion. "Ya wanna go back home to Pittsburgh with me?" he asked.

"Wow, I'd love to!" Lie! It was the last place I wanted to go!

"Hi, I'm Kris, Brian's girlfriend."

"So nice to meet you, Kris, you know Brian was the big man on campus."

"Yes, I've heard."

"You must be really special, what do you do for a living?"

"Cancer."

I was a nervous wreck. But since Brian was my Steve McQueen, my badass-fuck-cancer-and-live-on-the-edge man, it was the least I could do. We started dating after my diagnosis, which earned him major points as a stand-up guy. Brian drove a motorcycle and owned a yoga mat. He listened to Bob Dylan and read Alan Watts. He was my dream man.

The members of his high school gang were still pretty tight. In fact, they called themselves "the bubble." All outsiders who marry into the bubble (male or female) were called "bubble wives," a title that caused me great concern.

Because the bubble people knew I was sick, I was determined to look the opposite—drop-dead gorgeous. I resurrected a really short skirt, push-up bra, tight top, and pink heels for the occasion. Sex Kitten Barbie was the look I was going for, and I was successful. I even upstaged the prom queen.

The night was amazing. By 2:00 a.m. I was holding court in the ladies' room with my gaggle of new bubble BFFs. We even made a 5:00 a.m. trip to Permanny Brothers for some greasy fries (a tasty treat that was galaxies away from my "healing diet"). The boys had tipped back one too many libations while reminiscing about "the good ol' days," so I played chauffeur in Brian's pickup truck. Did I mention it's a stick shift? Needless to say, I passed the cool-girlfriend test with flying colors. The next day he told me (through his hangover haze) how proud he was to have such an amazing girl in his life. Mission accomplished!

94

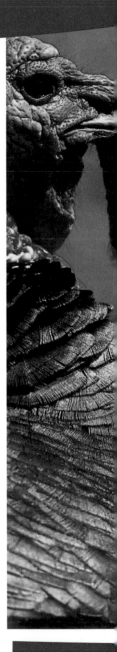

tip no.47

CREATE A CODE WORD— *turkey!*

Code words signal your partner to cease and desist when the conversation gets too tough. This may sound silly, but couples have been using this technique during kinky sex for generations. Why? Because when we explore the unknown, we need to do it with a flashlight and a bulletproof vest! I use the word *turkey*. Unfortunately, Brian and I learned this trick the hard way.

All went swimmingly at the reunion. But the big drive home was a big disaster. With no radio and a seven-hour trip ahead of us, we had plenty of time to talk about everything . . . and I mean everything. Childhood memories, first loves, arrests, and of course cancer. We tried to corral our imaginations. But they bucked

and reared, sending us galloping through a deep exploration of the "what-ifs." Brian is a pretty stoic and private guy who never likes to burden people with his problems. Plus, the thought of sharing his emotions makes him feel, as he says, "a little fruity."

So in keeping with my new cool-girlfriend status, I gave him the go-ahead to mind-dump. "Don't hold back, you need to let it out, I can take it." He cringed and reluctantly shared some of his fears. I was surprised at how well I listened (a skill I was still trying to master). But then out of nowhere, I got a wild itchin' to know his big-picture intentions. So against my better judgment, I fished and I pried. With only twenty-four hours until the big move-in,

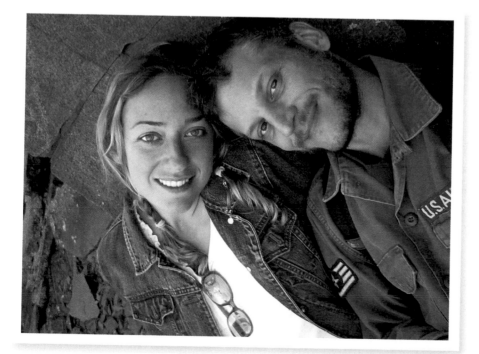

the timing couldn't have been worse. "Do you want to marry me?" I asked. We demanded that our relationship be open and honest, so he felt it was safe to be truthful. He had no idea he was about to walk into a turkey.

"Well, we'll see, let's take it slow. I'm happy right now, but I'm not sure I see this working for the long haul."

"Huh?"

"To be honest, sometimes I think that staying single gives me a way out if things get bad."

"What?"

"I'm afraid of being totally drained and incapable of dealing with the potential hard times."

"You're afraid!?"

"Plus, I want kids, and since you may not be able to have them I really need to think about that."

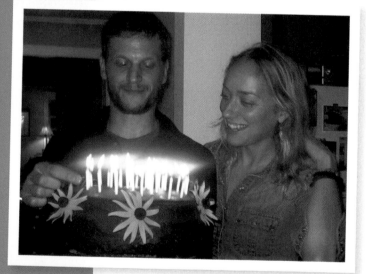

"TURKEY!"

I burst into tears and cried the rest of the way home. If he wanted safe, he could go find a boring mediocre girl! If he wanted fabulous, even if only for fifteen minutes, then I was his gal. Though he apologized five hundred times, nothing but whiskey could make me feel better. Of course he had a right to his feelings. Who wouldn't question the future when falling in love with a cancer patient? (Oops, I mean survivor!) But the thought of losing him because of my stupid disease made me feel trapped and furious. The next day all my boxes arrived. He kissed me, apologized seven more times, and went to work. I just sat there, numb. There I was, in his space, surrounded by my boxes and emotional shrapnel.

It's hard when your imagination takes you on a tour of your coffin. It's even harder when someone else's does. TURKEY! If you can't go there, don't. Establish psychological boundaries and suggest your partner get additional support. Also, don't dig. And put a moratorium on the dark fantasies: They do nothing but wreak havoc!

Co-survivors often feel a deep sense of helplessness. The fear of losing Marvelous You can be overwhelming, so it's important for them to have a safe place (like a shrink's office) to voice their feelings. Be willing to talk, but protect yourself. Try as you might, it's not always easy for either of you to remain objective.

chapter four in review:

remember:

You are a survivor the day you are diagnosed!

The time to start taking risks and planning for your future is now.

Make a list of ten things you've always wanted to do and try them.

We can change the trajectory of our lives no matter what seemingly insurmountable obstacles stand in our way.

Tap into your artistic mojo.

Journaling is an inexpensive way to give yourself therapy.

Going on a retreat or getaway of any kind can help you reflect and process all the changes cancer has made in your life.

Seek out the healer within yourself.

Custom-design a spiritual practice that works for you—but only if that works for you!

Don't forget the pain that your co-survivors, your Crazy Sexy Cancer Angels, are experiencing. Tell them how grateful you are.

Make time to be present for your co-survivors.

Establish psychological boundaries with your partner. Suggest that he or she get additional support.

Turkey!

CHAPTER FIVE

go ahead— USE THE CANCER CARD

Congratulations! You have been preapproved for a Platinum Club Cancer Card membership! Though it sucks that you have cancer (and we're very sorry about that), membership to this ever-growing club does come with its perks. Your Cancer Card provides you with oodles of mileage points and has no expiration date. It's an I'm-human card, and like it or not you can't do it all; every now and then you need a treat.

Sometimes just knowing that your card is available in a pinch or on a rainy cancer day can really put your mind at ease.

Here are a few club rules to keep in mind: (1) Your membership begins the day you are diagnosed. (2) It is nontransferable. (3) There is no annual charge, interest rate, or debt. (4) You may swipe your card freely, but we urge you to use some discretion. Tragically, the card can be declined. Therefore, as with all major credit cards, make sure you take the time to read the fine print!

HOSPITAL OVERNIGHT STAY:
$10,000

CUSTOM WIG:
$1,500–6,000

OUT-OF-POCKET MEDICATION COSTS:
$3,000

USE OF YOUR CANCER CARD TO GET OUT OF BRUNCH WITH YOUR BOSS AND HER KIDS:
Priceless.

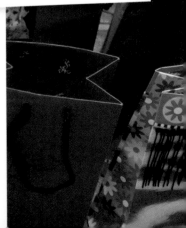

tip no.48

USE IT, *don't abuse it!*

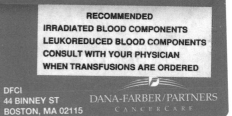

ALWAYS BRING THIS CARD WITH YOU

RECOMMENDED
IRRADIATED BLOOD COMPONENTS
LEUKOREDUCED BLOOD COMPONENTS
CONSULT WITH YOUR PHYSICIAN
WHEN TRANSFUSIONS ARE ORDERED

DFCI
44 BINNEY ST
BOSTON, MA 02115

DANA-FARBER/PARTNERS
C A N C E R C A R E

On my first day at the Dana-Farber Cancer Institute, I was given a little blue plastic card that changed my life. "Here's your new ID card, Kris. Please bring it with you EVERYWHERE, FOREVER." No turning back now, I thought, I'm in the system. For a broad who likes to keep under the radar (you never know when you'll need an alibi), this was totally invasive! With just one swipe my stats were on display for all the cancer world to see. It amazed me how a tiny piece of plastic could add about a thousand pounds of emotional weight to my wallet. But because I wanted to be a "good" cancer patient, I obeyed and took the card with me everywhere. One time I even pulled it out at the lingerie counter at Bloomingdale's. It must have been wrestling for top wallet slot, a spot my Amex card generally gets. Boy, did that cause a stir. There's nothing worse than obtusely checking your "crackberry" while the cashier is loudly sounding out "Dana-Farber Cancer Institute." "Sorry, baby, we don't take this card here. But do you mind if I ask you a question? Are you in remission yet?" Yet? Keep the panties, I'm outta here!

When I first started swiping my card, I thought the skies would open and a bolt of lightning would strike me in the ass. "No I can't do the dishes, I have cancer." BOOM! OUCH! KARMIC EXPLOSION! My husband has even warned me, "Don't use cancer as an excuse to get out of stuff unless it's for real. Remember the tale about the boy who cried wolf?" Point taken. Use it, don't abuse it. Because when the imaginary magnetic strip wears out, that's it, no replacements.

There are any number of perfectly valid reasons to swipe your Cancer Card. For further information regarding member privileges and limitations, read on.

swipe for an OUT, *or an* IN

This is a vital way to use the card, especially for the ladies who have a hard time voicing their needs. When you carry the Cancer Card, you automatically become a VIP, top-priority client. Members do not have to wait in long lines or get dragged to football games, baby or wedding showers, brunches, happy hours, et cetera.

- I need to rest. *I have cancer.*

- Don't dump your garbage on me. *I have cancer!*

- I regret to inform you that due to *cancer*, I will not be able to attend your party.

- I can't come to work today. *I have cancer* (plus I'll miss Oprah).

- I have to cut this conversation short (you toxic blabbermouth), I'm not feeling so hot. (A subtle way of saying *The cancer is acting up.*)

swipe away for
CANCER TANTRUMS

Sometimes we're well-behaved citizens who happen to have cancer. Other times we're irrational lunatics WITH CANCER! swinging wildly on a speeding pendulum between rage and tears. If you need to explain your behavior in the aftermath of a huge meltdown, just pull out the Cancer Card.

- Oh my word, I have no idea why I behaved that way! Really it wasn't me, it was the cancer!

- I don't have to deal with this nonsense, I have cancer!

- No you can't have that parking spot, I have cancer! Back off!

swipe for
SHOPPING THERAPY

(More about shopping therapy below.)

- I have nothing to wear and I have cancer? (That just ain't right.)

- I have to have scans so I want to reward myself with something new.

FAUX PAS!

Remember, just because you have cancer doesn't mean you won't have to apologize at times. The Cancer Card can't get you out of taking responsibility for when your emotions push you too far and hurt someone.

- I had scans so I want to reward myself with something new.

- I hate scans so I want to reward myself with something new.

- I blew off my scans so I want to reward myself with something new.

- I'm blue, I need something new.

- My apartment needs some feng shui for healing, I'd better get something new.

- I'm fat, I need something new.

- I'm skinny . . . the list is endless!

tip no.49

BROWSING BOOSTS
your immune system

Have you ever heard the phrase *shopping high*? Well, it's an actual physical state caused by the release of high levels of serotonin and dopamine into your system. These mood-lifting drugs are the same chemicals released when eating chocolate bonbons or falling head over heels in love! Okay, so I'm not a scientist, but it all seems pretty straightforward to me. Who

hasn't felt that surging level of ecstasy created by finding the perfect pair of jeans that makes your butt super-fabulous? Don't you just laugh out loud in delight? On top of the sheer feeling of joy when you score such a purchase, studies have shown that there is a strong relationship between the brain and the immune system, and that happiness actually boosts your ability to fight disease. So grab your Cancer Card and your Amex card!

In times of duress there's no better prescription than a little retail therapy. I don't care if it's Saks or Target, a few laps around a department store can really lift your spirits. You don't even have to make a purchase; the art of surveying is equally powerful. Remember those old Calgon bubble bath commercials? The ones where a tired, stressed model would bellow, "Calgon, take me away!" Well, that's exactly what a little shopping therapy can do for you—take you away from the stress of your life into a world of baubles, fashion, a new perfume, a box of sinful chocolates. Or homey items to coz-i-fy your pad. Sometimes finding just the right curtains to keep the world out while you go in can make all the difference.

Plus, let's face it, shopping is a sport.

You can play it alone or with a team (your posse). And if you're really serious about it, I suggest a good pair of sneakers (New Balance is my brand of choice). Why not kill two birds with one stone and get a workout, too? It is helpful to do a little pregame gam stretch before you take off. There's nothing worse than a carpe diem cancer shopping spree cut short by the crippling effects of crampy mall legs. Even when I just wander aimlessly taking in all the visual stimuli in the shops, I leave in a better mood.

Looking and feeling good is important to gals dealing with the surgeries and side effects of cancer treatments. Whether the changes are noticeable or not, the psychological effects can do a number on the ol' self-esteem. Finding clothing and accessories to cover a port, expanders, different-size breasts, a colostomy

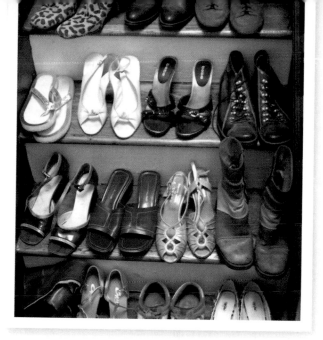

bag, or even just a really depressed mood can help salvage some sense of dignity and control.

Don't worry about what you had or what you lost; accentuate the positive! Dress your personality and for God's sake accessorize! A life without trinkets is tragic.

Think colors, too. Don't just go for funeral black (unless of course you live in New York City—then, like it or not, black is your uniform). Colors can really brighten your mood and your style. I adore emerald green—it makes my eyes pop and my complexion look great. It's also the color of the heart chakra, symbolizing harmony, creativity, health, and abundance—rock on! If you're interested, there are many books on the healing power of color. Lots of gals I know apply color therapy to their wardrobes and even their wigs. Why not? If red is your color, then paint the town! Just be wary of going overboard. You don't want to look like a cross between a Christmas tree and Bozo the Clown.

PLAY CANCER
dress-up

When I was little, I used to love to watch my mom get dressed for a date with my dad. It was fascinating, like witnessing a sacred ritual filled with perfumes, pretty jewels, lovely dresses, and groovy purses. I'd wait until the coast was clear and then raid her closet, exploring what I'd look like all grown up and fancy. Twenty-five years later I grab my best gal and raid a much bigger retail closet in my game of cancer dress-up. Even if you aren't quite ready to embrace the looks of the new you, you may find some pleasure in shopping for her. Just remember that all therapies have their limits—and so does your cash flow.

FAUX PAS!

Bankruptcy is *not* therapeutic. Cancer isn't an excuse to become an ST addict. According to the American Psychological Association, an estimated fifteen million Americans are compulsive shoppers, meaning they can't control how much they shop. Some 90 percent of compulsive shoppers are women. I bet most of those gals are Cancer Babes! Though you deserve caviar and emotional cashmere, keep your budget in perspective and save the retail therapy for times you really need a lift. Leaving the house with a vague idea, a panic attack, and a Visa card can be a recipe for disaster. Why not explore thrift stores, the Salvation Army, flea markets, garage sales . . . ST doesn't have to be a big high-roller blow-out. It's simply an attitude adjustment.

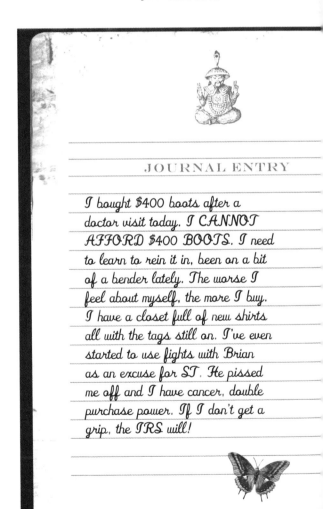

JOURNAL ENTRY

I bought $400 boots after a doctor visit today. I CANNOT AFFORD $400 BOOTS. I need to learn to rein it in, been on a bit of a bender lately. The worse I feel about myself, the more I buy. I have a closet full of new shirts all with the tags still on. I've even started to use fights with Brian as an excuse for ST. He pissed me off and I have cancer, double purchase power. If I don't get a grip, the IRS will!

{ best shopping therapy purchase, best swipe, and worst DECLINE! }

In a stitch-and-bitch-like fashion, I asked members of my posse to share their best shopping therapy purchase, best wiggle-my-way-into- or out-of-something swipe, and worst DECLINE! Here's what these fabulous Cancer Babes, myself included, had to say:

Heidi

BEST S.T. PURCHASE I wasn't big on shopping while I was in treatment, mostly because I wasn't thrilled with the way I looked, and those three-way mirrors and the fitting room lighting only made me feel worse. So my shopping therapy took the form of plane tickets. I planned trips as interim goals to look forward to during my year-plus of treatment, and it made a big difference in my mental health.

BEST SWIPE I used my Cancer Card more to get things than to get out of things. I reserved using my card for moments like jumping to the front of lines or making my brothers do things for me.

DECLINED! I tried to get down to the floor level to be closer to the stage at an Eagles concert at Texas Stadium. No luck!

CancerVixen

Marisa

BEST S.T. PURCHASE I really needed rain boots, so I splurged and bought a pair by Pucci! I thought, If I'm going to tramp out to treatment in the rain I might as well be wearing something I love. My mother also gave me a pink fur hat. I would wear it on the days when I had radiation; when I walked into the center, people would laugh. Not only was I curing myself, I was curing other people as well. That pink fur hat was pretty sassy.

BEST SWIPE While I was getting chemo, I would tell my cartoonist friends to call me at a certain time. When they did, we would have funny conversations and they would make me laugh. When I told them what I was doing, they would get really uncomfortable. I was like, No, don't feel bad, you're part of the therapy, you help the chemo by putting a smile on my face.

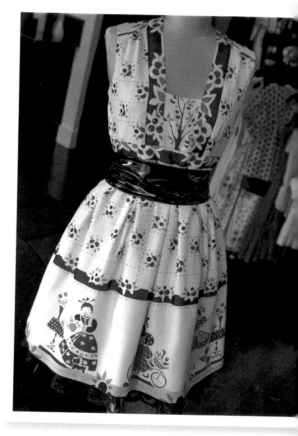

DECLINED! One of my BFFs, Sharon, was having a baby shower. She had been trying to get pregnant for a while, so the shower wasn't just a run-of-the-mill party, it was meant to be a real celebration. I had a round of chemo treatments two days before the shower was scheduled, and my white cell count was really low; I had also gotten this really awful shot that felt like I had had cement injected in my veins. So when Sharon called me and said, "You're coming to my shower, right?" I pulled out my Cancer Card: "Sharon, I just got my shot, and I just got my treatment, and they told me if I don't have to do something then I really shouldn't." She replied, "Oh that's really terrible! What time will you be here?" So my card was DECLINED!

Erin

BEST S.T. PURCHASE Every six months I travel to Portland for a bone marrow biopsy. After the procedure I always treat myself to some shopping therapy and a beer. The first of these shopping therapy sessions involved a $350 Coach bag, which is a lot of money to me. I'm not one to splurge; it took my mom's gentle coaxing to persuade me to buy the bag. But there is something to be said for dropping a lot of cash, especially when you no longer feel like yourself. It's a rush, and it feels good, and you end up with a nice collection of accessories. The best part of my retail therapy is that it enables me to take control of the experience by making it positive. Instead of "I went to Portland and had all this cancer stuff done and it was a drag," it's "I went to Portland and look what a great bag I scored!"

BEST SWIPE I got out of jury duty indefinitely, which I'd say is pretty darn good. But in general I use my Cancer Card less to get out of things and more to give me permission to do things, like eat french fries or buy expensive bags or sleep ten hours a night.

DECLINED! My card is declined by my husband, Nick, on a regular basis. He just doesn't pity me in any way shape or form, which is, of course, why I love him. He'll do things for me, like clean the kitchen, the bathroom, do the laundry, et cetera, because he loves me, not because I have cancer. Anytime I try to play that card, he rolls his eyes. I am, after all, perfectly healthy.

Melissa

BEST S.T. PURCHASE Two days after I was diagnosed, I bought a pair of Chanel sunglasses and a Coach diaper bag. I figured if I was going to be a bald mom, I would at least be a well-accessorized bald mom!

BEST SWIPE During the three years I was a cancer patient, I went to about fifteen weddings. At each one, I would tell everyone at my table that I had cancer and I wanted the centerpiece. No one ever objected. Except of course my husband, who had to carry them out when we left.

DECLINED! Because I have to share my Cancer Card with my sister, who also has cancer, it carries less weight with my family, where it's regularly DECLINED!

Lindsay

BEST S.T. PURCHASE I continued to pay rent on my New York City apartment while I was getting treatment and living at home in San Francisco. That apartment represented my freedom at the end of it all. Having it meant I could go back to my life.

BEST SWIPE I use my Cancer Card most to get better medical treatments. For example, I hate needles and pain, so I know how to swipe my card to improve my experience. With in vitro fertilization, I managed to get morphine after a procedure when everyone else was getting Tylenol!

DECLINED! I've yet to be DECLINED!

Suzanne

BEST S.T. PURCHASE I've always been a big saver, but when I received my diagnosis I started to look at things just a tad differently. Why not live life to the fullest? Why not buy the boat that my husband had been talking about incessantly? Putting the down payment on the damn boat became a way of af-firming that I was going to get through it! We took our first ride the day before I started chemo. It felt so wonderful putting my face in the sun and being out on the ocean, nothing else mattered!

BEST SWIPE Last fall I was forced to turn down a position with a stock photo agency. At the time, I concluded it was best for me to stay put. However, I recently used my Cancer Card to reopen communications.

DECLINED! After an initial response, that potential employer has not followed through getting back to me!

FAUX PAS!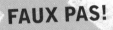

Beware of Cancer Card theft! Situations might arise where others may try to use your Cancer Card on you. I had one friend who used to guilt me into calling her back by leaving really pushy and inappropriate messages on my machine. "I've called several times, you're really starting to worry me. Are you okay? If you don't call me back, you know what I'll think. Please be considerate and call." Give me a break! If I were dead you'd be the first person I'd tell.

Sharon

BEST S.T. PURCHASE A gift package of massage treatments at Bliss spa (yummmm!).

BEST SWIPE A few years ago, when I was still undergoing

treatment, I was rushing to get from my mom's house in North Miami to Gilda's Club in Fort Lauderdale to take a yoga class. It was rush hour and the traffic was tight, so I was speeding and went into the carpool lane, which requires two passengers, and got pulled over! The officer asked me where I was going in such a hurry and why was I in the carpool lane. I told him that I had just finished a chemotherapy treatment and needed to get to my yoga class (it was the truth, but I just blurted it out before my brain could process it). He took off his hat and sunglasses (soooo Miami!), knelt down, and looked at me for a very long five seconds. I just stared back at him. Finally he gave me back my license and paperwork, and told me to stay out of the carpool lane and to have a nice day.

DECLINED! I was buying a wig to use for a short film I was shooting and came across a place that offered discounts to cancer patients. The woman at the counter asked for proof that I was a cancer patient! I asked her if anyone had ever really lied about having cancer to get a 20 percent discount on a wig. She stared back at me, completely blank, and without a scrap of emotion again asked for proof of my cancer. I didn't have my "cancer papers" or my cancer ID badge or my I-HAD-CANCER-AND-ALL-I-GOT-WAS-THIS-LOUSY-T-SHIRT tee on. I was stunned and flustered. When I showed her my eight-inch scar, she said that I could have been pregnant and had a C-section. I pointed out the irony of having a discount set up for such a compassionate and beautiful reason and totally shitting on it by her behavior. I then remembered that I had a letter from Sloan-Kettering confirming my consultation appointment in my bag. I showed it to her and left—sans wig, pride intact.

Jackie

BEST S.T. PURCHASE A new bed that I love. It happens to be the exact model used in the Four Seasons hotels. Works for me.

BEST SWIPE I still haven't broken out my Cancer Card. I do think about breaking it out and would use it if I felt the situation warranted it. I better do something soon because I plan on cutting the card up very soon!

Allison

| BEST S.T. PURCHASE | After I finished chemo and my first surgery, I booked myself a "healing retreat" in Hawaii. I vowed to spend the entire vacation healing my mind, body, and spirit. I figured I owed it to myself after what I had been through. I spent my first week with my best friend from childhood, Jen. The second week I stayed at a wellness center. By the time I returned home, I felt like a new woman! I also decided to spoil myself with new bedding. I figured if I was going to have to spend a lot of time sick in bed, then I wanted it to be really nice. My bed is now so soft and comfy. I've nicknamed it "clouds of heaven."

| BEST SWIPE | Taking a year off from work and allowing people to take care of me. I am a very independent and driven person, so neither of these things was easy to accept at first. However, once I adjusted, I realized how nice it was to spend my days doing only the things that mattered (I didn't have the energy for much else!). It really put things into perspective. Cancer is not an easy experience, but it does provide an opportunity for a lot of self-growth and discovery. The Cancer Card gives you the opportunity to look within and reflect and to focus on only what you have in the "now."

| DECLINED! | For me, the Cancer Card got declined when I realized that it was time for my life to go back to "normal." I couldn't stay in my world of doctor's appointments and disability checks forever. It's more like my Cancer Card expired. Now I carry the "survivor card." It's in my back pocket at all times and, whenever life hits a bump, I whip it out and remind myself to put things into perspective.

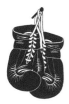

Terri

| BEST S.T. PURCHASE | The best thing I bought myself was time. I stopped being such a workaholic and made the gym a priority. I always went but wasn't strict about it. I would give it up for other obligations. A.C. (After Cancer) I decided that the gym was non-negotiable. Other things could wait and did. To this day I go to the gym five to six days a week.

BEST SWIPE I was involved with a financial group that I had long wanted to get out of and absolutely used my Cancer Card to bail hard-core.

DECLINED! I got up the gumption to confront a friend about her disappearing act during my ordeal. I was like, "If you have issues with your own mortality, that's not my problem blah blah blah." I realized by the expression on her face that she had either forgotten I had cancer or just really "wasn't that into me." So that made my Cancer Card null and void. Our friendship ended right then and there—imagine that!

Diem

BEST S.T. PURCHASE The best thing I bought with my Cancer Card was the Web site for my organization, Live for the Challenge. In fact, through my Web site's medical gift registry, the family and friends of a Cancer Babe can actually chip in for her retail therapy!

Here's how the idea for my Web site came to me. One day I was sitting at my computer feeling depressed because I was having a hard time paying for my prescriptions and trying to figure out how to pay for a real-looking wig. I went to check my e-mail and was bombarded by messages from my "healthy" friends who were twenty-something southern belles busy getting married and having babies. Waiting in my inbox were messages directing me to their baby and wedding registries.

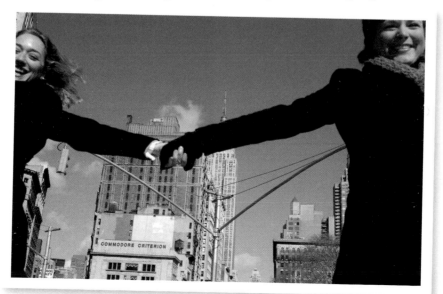

Me and Diem

And that's when the idea hit me: We celebrate the birth of a life with a baby registry; the joining of two lives with a wedding registry; but there is no registry for the fight for a life. I decided then and there to create a medical gift registry for people dealing with illness.

Here's how it works: Folks battling an illness select items they need via the online registry, and their loved ones are then able to purchase those items for them and send them as gifts. Anyone can go to the registry and help out with things that someone who is battling illness might need—groceries, maid service, in-home care, assistance with household needs and upkeep, educational assistance, babysitting/driving/pet care services, a little spa treatment, a plane ticket, a wig, or even just the conventional flowers and a pick-me-up card.

BEST SWIPE I didn't want to feel any different from my friends and family, so I honestly never used it. But ooohhh what I would do with that card now!

DECLINED! Ew, that happens?!

Jodi

BEST S.T. PURCHASE My shoe collection. I actually reached a point where I felt as though I couldn't buy another pair of shoes! I did a lot of online shopping. Packages would arrive that I didn't remember ordering because I was so whacked out on drugs at the time. Every day was Christmas!

BEST SWIPE I am the Cancer Card Queen! I am absolutely shameless and hope that I am not damned to hell as a result. I've swiped it to get free hotel rooms, board airplanes early, not wait in line, get special discounts, get free tickets and preferred seats, special meals, free drinks . . . the list goes on. I've used it as an excuse for not having to do just about anything and to get out of every type of social obligation.

DECLINED! Surprisingly infrequently! In recent memory, only when I tried to use it to get the interest rate on my credit card lowered.

Me

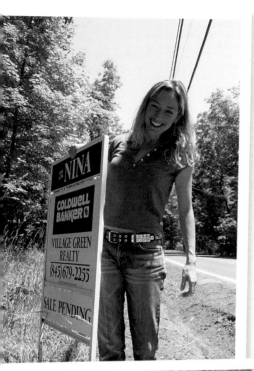

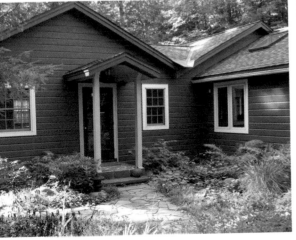

BEST S.T. PURCHASE Remember how I used to find my personal refuge on mountain walks in Woodstock, New York? Well, the healing wood nymphs encouraged me to relocate. Screw cancer, hello debt and mortgage! Of course, cancer tried to dampen the big day for me, but I refused to let it. My unknowing Realtor revealed (in a hushed tone) that the previous owner had died of cancer. "How lucky are we to have our health?" she uttered. Yeah, yeah, show me the bedroom. That annoying incident aside, the purchase was exhilarating! Owning a house with four walls and an acre can make you feel like such a grown-up. It may sound old-fashioned, but my marriage and that house have made me feel that the future has an anchor.

BEST SWIPE I recently joined a gym only to avoid it. Not only that, I signed up for ten nonrefundable boxing sessions with an ex-Olympian. What was I thinking? After three sessions I was shredded! Though I did get a lot of anger out, it took me weeks to recover. I even told my trainer, "I have cancer so I can't do five thousand crunches or my liver will fall out." He didn't give a damn. For my own safety I decided to quit. When I told the manager that I wanted my money back, he said no way no how. I had no choice but to invoke the Cancer Card! "Sir, I'm about to start a very dangerous clinical trial for cancer and the last thing I need to do is come here and get my ass kicked. What can you do for me?" Well, I didn't get a refund, but I did get each remaining session transferred to a massage. Now we're talking!

DECLINED! My film was rejected by a network whose name I shall not mention. Apparently cancer was "just too hard a sell with a less-than-narrow viewer base." I found that pretty hard to believe, especially since about 1.4 million people will be diagnosed in this country this year alone. It was shocking to me that an uplifting story about survival would get lost in the shuffle of celebrity poker, tattoos, and cellulite removal shows. But alas, I was DECLINED!

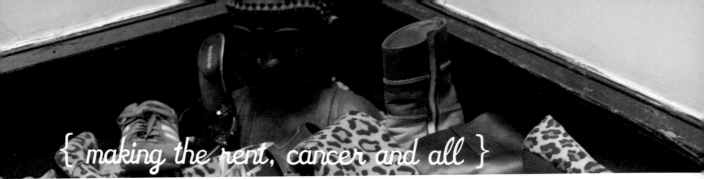

{ making the rent, cancer and all }

Unfortunately, the Cancer Card does have its limitations. It won't cover the rent, your mortgage, or your utility bills, and it won't stock your pantry with organic, all-natural groceries. Many women have to, and want to, work during and after treatment. But being on your game and maintaining your image and energy at the office can be challenging. You may need breaks, naps, sick days, or a desk that's close to the bathroom! Some women simply can't work during treatment. It's im-portant to know your limits and research your options for financial assistance. Explore the possibility of qualifying for disability or asking for a loan from your family. You can even plan a fund-raiser. Get creative and strategize your grassroots save-my-toosh-from-the-poorhouse campaign! I have several friends who had par-ties and events to offset their out-of-pocket medical expenses and their day-to-day costs like rent and chow. If it makes you feel weird, have someone else host it.

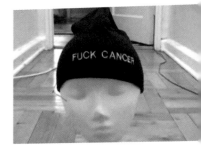

{ a little help from friends }

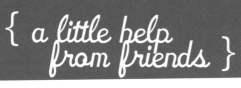

My Cancer Posse pal Jackie Farry threw an awesome benefit concert called "Fuck Cancer" (my sentiments exactly) to help pay for her medical expenses and the time off she'd have to take from her hectic job as a rock-and-roll tour manager. You may remember Jackie from the MTV show *Superock*—she was the hip host! While on the road with one of her bands in the winter of 2003, Jackie was diagnosed with multiple myeloma, a rare blood cancer. With little insurance, no work, and a pile of medical bills, Jackie created the Fuck Cancer Benefit Concert and Raffle. In an effort to creatively raise money, she asked her music pals to help out. Ask and ye shall receive! The show sold out. It was mind blowing how many amazing people donated prizes. Guitars, drum lessons, magazine subscriptions, autographed CDs by famous celebrities, even a vintage *Playboy* collection!

PROFILE:
JACKIE FARRY

AGE: 40 (on paper)

HAIR COLOR: Brown

EYES: Brown

HEIGHT: 5'3"-ish. I shrank about an inch and a half from my cancer.

WEIGHT: Have you ever been on steroids for more than a year? I gained 20 pounds in the first month of my latest treatment. On a positive note, the chemo/roid combo actually worked. Fat and in remission.

HOMETOWN: New York

OCCUPATION: Tour-managing rock bands—however, fighting cancer is my full-time job at the moment.

FAVORITE SAYING: "Fuck cancer!"

BEST TIP: When you're recovering, try not to beat yourself up. If you're having a bad day either physically or emotionally and all you manage to do that day is walk your dog, that's okay. Set small, realistic goals and reward yourself when you meet them.

Jackie:

At first I felt uncomfortable asking others for help. But my bills just kept piling up. There was no way I could go back to work. I could barely function! So I got creative. I took the "fuck cancer" attitude right from the start, so I thought it would be a fitting name for my benefit. I organized two shows, one in New York and one in Los Angeles. I asked some of my favorite bands to play for free (another thing that was hard for me to do). Thanks to their efforts and the generosity of so many people who donated prizes and services, both shows were sold out and totally successful!

Everyone who performed took time out of their busy schedule to help me out of the shitty situation I was in. Being a tour manager, I knew that whenever a band I worked with played a benefit it was usually a big pain in the ass, no matter how worthwhile the cause. Having that insight made me feel even luckier. From the two shows—after expenses and donations to other young adult cancer charities—I cleared close to $20,000! The money helped me pay for my ever-increasing health insurance, my apartment, my commute back and forth to doctor's appointments, and food.

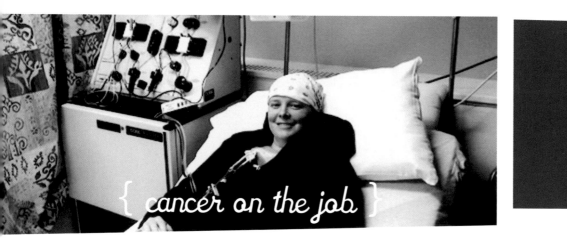

8)

Jackie Farry Fuck Cancer Benefit featuring the Jon Spencer Blues Explosion + Chavez + Har Mar Superstar + Quintron and Miss Pussycat + Cat Power + J Mascis (Bowery Ballroom, Tue 11) See "Beat box," page 119.

veteran band ith nton.

MUSIC

pest fs, it's t

The Stills (Irving Plaza, Tue 11) These young

I actually met Jackie at her benefit. Earlier that day I had been flipping through *Time Out* magazine when I came across the ad for the event. It was the coolest party I had been to post-diagnosis, and Jackie was so gracious. She let me film the entire event, which subsequently became the first day of filming two years of Jackie's life for my film. I'll never forget what a rush I felt standing in front of the crowd at the party thanking them for taking the time to come out and lifting my glass to fuck cancer!

{ cancer on the job }

Some women, like my friend Melissa, continue to plug away at their day jobs—cancer and all. Melissa is Erin's older sister. Within months of Erin's diagnosis of chronic myelogenous leukemia, Melissa found out she had Hodgkin's disease. She was seven months' pregnant at the time but had to start treatment right away. Thankfully, baby and mother are doing just fine, but what a way to start your life as a new mom! One of the things I find so inspiring about Melissa is her unstoppable can-do attitude. She is a cancer marine! Melissa is a take-no-prisoners CPA. I remember visiting her while she was checked into the hospital for an extended stay. It was the height of tax season, and that girl had a mobile office set up in her hospital room. To listen to her bark orders on the phone, you'd never know she was lying in a bed strapped to tubes. Whenever I have to suck it up, I think of that image of Melissa and pull myself up by my bootstraps.

melissa's icon:

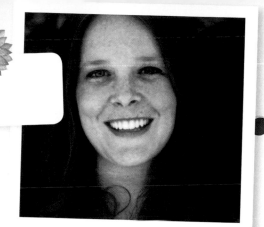

PROFILE:
MELISSA GONZALEZ

AGE: 30

HAIR COLOR: Flaming red
(before and after chemo)

EYES: Blue

HEIGHT: 5'7"

WEIGHT: Are you crazy! Thanks to cancer, too much to put in writing!

HOMETOWN: Huntington, New York

OCCUPATION: Certified public accountant

FAVORITE SAYING: "Everything happens for a reason."

BEST TIP: Life is short . . . enjoy it. No matter what it throws at you.

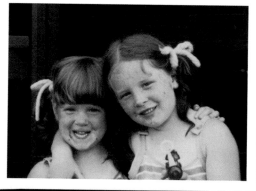

Melissa:

I was on maternity leave during my first treatment. Not really the way you want to spend your first weeks with your newborn, but I really didn't have a choice. After my three months of maternity leave were up, I went back to work. I still had daily radiation treatments to deal with, but my firm was very understanding. Still, they didn't pay me for the time I wasn't there, so money was tight. Because I could earn more working part time than I could collecting disability, I would work half a day, walk five minutes to the train station, take the thirty-

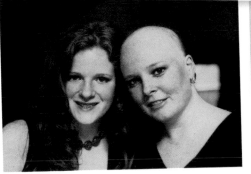

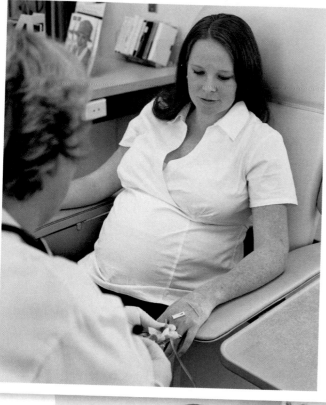

minute train ride from East Williston to Penn Station, jump on the subway, take the subway for twenty minutes to get as close to Sloan as I could, and then walk the remaining fifteen minutes to Sloan. I get tired just thinking of it, but I didn't want to pay the $15 cab fare or deal with the traffic, so that was my routine. I did this for twenty days and then was back to work full time.

Fast-forward nine months to when I found out my cancer was back and I would need a stem cell transplant. That go-round I was out of work for two months. And because it was tax season, I took my laptop to the hospital with me and did work when I had to. This time my firm paid me. I was extremely lucky.

We had just bought a house, and disability wouldn't even cover the cost of my son's formula, let alone the mortgage. I had a good relationship with my boss, and he was aware of our financial situation. He made the decision to pay me for the time I was out. Even so, I felt compelled to go back to work way before my doctor advised. I went to work with my mask and gloves on and closed my office door, hoping I wouldn't pick up any germs. The days when I was too weak or not feeling well, I would work from my laptop at home. Like most women these days, I felt I didn't have a choice.

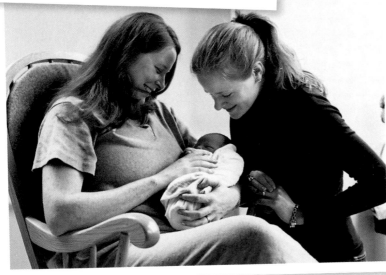

One salary does not cover the cost of living on Long Island, and disability pays nothing. My family had enough to worry about without having to pay our bills. Plus, I didn't mind the distraction work gave me. Lying in bed watching bad TV only made me feel like I was sick. I wanted to feel normal, and knowing my firm needed me helped me feel that way. I am happy to say that transplant and all, none of my clients went on extension that year.

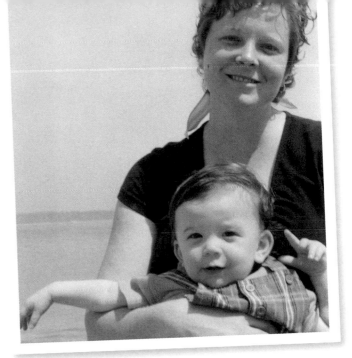

PROFILE:
ALLISON BRIGGS

allison's icon:

AGE: 27 (diagnosed at 26)

HAIR COLOR: Blond

EYES: Hazel

HEIGHT: 5′7″

WEIGHT: 110

HOMETOWN: San Diego, California

OCCUPATION: Real estate sales

FAVORITE SAYING: "What you think about, you bring about."

BEST TIP: Try to free your mind of attachments, expectations, and fear. Remember that it's the unexpected challenges that deliver us to better things.

{ taking a break }

Some women, like my friend Allison, actually have a positive experience with disability. When Alli was diagnosed with breast cancer, her mom, a cancer co-survivor and Alli's designated angel, took the burden of researching her financial options and dealing with her insurance so that Alli could focus on her recovery. Alli's mom Googled her way to the Web site for California disability insurance, which provided all the necessary information as well as a form to be completed. Alli's mom then helped her dig through her pay stubs to determine which quarter of the previous year's earnings information she wanted to submit—that is, when she'd made the most money. Once Alli had the form signed by her physician, she was good to go! She received her first check a month after submission.

> **"The truth will set you free. But first, it will piss you off."**
> **—GLORIA STEINEM,**
> **JOURNALIST AND ACTIVIST**

Allison:

When my doctor gave me the news of my breast cancer diagnosis and told me I had "Stage II infiltrating ductal carcinoma," all I could think was, *What does that mean?* I knew she was telling me I had cancer, but I had never known anyone with cancer before. All I could think was, *What is going to happen to my life? Will I have to quit my job? Will I have to move out of my town house?* I had no idea what cancer treatment entailed or what it would do to me physically.

The next day I met with my doctor again. I told her that I wanted to keep my life as intact as possible. I was hoping she would allow me to continue to work during my treatments. Well, this was completely out of the question (and as soon as I began chemo I learned why!). She told me that she would highly recommend that I take nine months off of work; I might even want to take a full year. That was a shock! She told me that I would be in chemo for three months, and it would leave me feeling tired and flu-like (as well as hairless). Then I would be having a bilateral mastec-

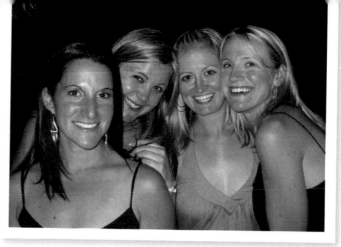

tomy, which would require a stay in the hospital followed by a few weeks' recoup time; then I would most likely begin radiation treatment, which would last another two months and also make me very tired. Following the radiation, I would finish my reconstructive surgery. She advised that I look into state disability leave.

I was diagnosed on November 30, 2005, and I had some vacation and sick leave accumulated with my employer. I decide to wait for January 1, 2006, to file a claim. Being on disability was great. It took so much stress off an already very stressful situation. I received a check every two weeks, always right on time, and I was lucky that the payments sustained my life (covered my rent, car payment, food, et cetera) and paid all my medical

ENLISTING UNCLE SAM'S HELP

It's possible that as a result of your diagnosis, you'll be able to receive Social Security disability benefits. To qualify, you will need to have been in the workforce for five out of ten years. However, younger workers—thirty-one years old or younger—can qualify with fewer years under their belts. For the most part, you qualify if you cannot do the work you did before your diagnosis. The Social Security Administration (SSA) will determine if you're eligible. In order to be considered, your disability must be expected to last for at least one year.

To apply, you'll need to complete an application for Social Security benefits and so-called Adult Disability Report. The report collects information about your condition and how it affects your ability to work. You can complete the forms online at www.ssa.gov/applyfordisability, or you can schedule an appointment with your local Social Security office. If your application is approved, you'll get your first full check the sixth full month after the date SSA deems that your disability began. Also, your children and spouse may receive benefits on your behalf.

How much will you be paid? That all depends on how much you've worked and earned in the past.

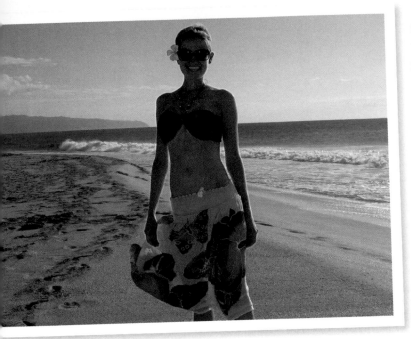

to other young women who are fighting cancer. The ultimate goal is to make the benefit an annual event.

In an article she wrote that appeared in *Self* magazine, my friend Oni talks about how she came to realize that the best thing she could do for herself was slow down and nurture her body.

Oni:

After my breast cancer diagnosis in 1996, when I was thirty-seven, my first thought was, I'm too busy to be sick! I'm a compulsively exercising, breast-feeding, breadwinning black mother of two. Who has time to have cancer! I convinced my medical team to perform my mastectomy and reconstructive surgery ASAP, so I could begin filming my first movie role in which I had more than one line. Shortly after the surgery, I hopped on a plane and flew to Toronto to film. During my chemo treatments, my doctors prescribed medications that mitigated chemo's side effects and adjusted my treatment schedule to accommodate my work. It all went well, and I got back into the swing of my busy life. Then in 1999 I had a reoccurrence. I did radiation, the doctors changed my medication and I kept on going. But in 2004, on the set of a television show I was working on, I became violently ill after filming wrapped. I actually had a seizure right in my trailer and had to be rushed to the hospital.

bills. Luckily, I had excellent medical insurance.

My efforts to pay it forward and help others fight their battles with cancer circled back and provided a supplement to my disability checks. Along with about a dozen close friends, I formed "The Rack Pack." The Rack Pack held various fund-raisers and built a Web site: www. therackpack.org.

During the course of our efforts, several people mentioned that they would like to contribute directly to my cause. We decided to add a donation button to the site to allow people to help with my medical expenses. We called it the Fight! Alli campaign. On top of that, we threw a benefit party for the Fight! Alli cause. Our goal was not only to help with my immediate financial needs, but also to create an ongoing effort to help other young women. We hope to throw another benefit this year and donate the proceeds

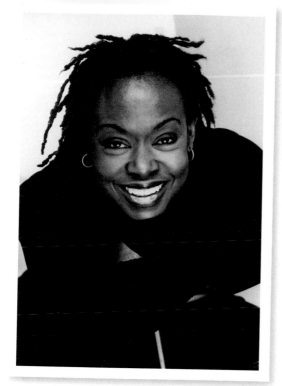

I ceased to be the do-it-all survivor. And then I felt ashamed: There was a "right" way of having cancer, and I was doing it wrong. No one blamed me, but I blamed myself. Over time, I let that go, too. I prayed, slept, cried and (don't tell anybody) felt sorry for myself, and—lo and behold, the roof didn't fall in! I wasn't instantly struck down! I washed one damn dish at a time, and when I was tired, I learned to stop. If making the bed took an hour and a half, so be it.

For me, being self-employed and an actress (like Oni) presented a whole different set of challenges. No security! Since I was a member

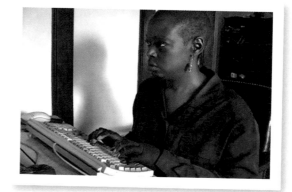

In the ER, a CAT scan revealed a few small brain tumors that had caused my seizure. I needed radiation. The eight-week recovery that followed forced me to sit down, shut up and stay home. I was weak, bald, swollen-faced and fragile, incapable of doing anything for the first time in my adult life. If I accomplished nothing, I thought, what right had I to survive? It felt like the end.

My body gave me no choice but to sit with those thoughts. No getting up and getting busy when I got scared. No shouting slogans ("I'm happy, healthy, whole and complete!") at myself. My brain refused to host the usual riot of self-punishing thoughts I'd mistaken for ambition, such as, "You're shit at the end of the day if you haven't done 13 things."

Perhaps the hardest part of this enforced stillness was my fear that those who loved me would be disappointed if

of the Screen Actors Guild, the acting union, I had great insurance—though I needed to earn a certain amount per year in TV or film or I'd lose it. And emotionally, I just couldn't deal with the bullshit of working in the entertainment industry. Yes, I wanted to be someone else, anyone else, but I was too preoccupied and scared to pretend in front of casting directors, advertisers, and network executives. Plus, in the beginning I didn't believe cancer was sexy for an unknown starlet battling to make a name for herself.

An average day pre-cancer for me was filled with tons of auditions and many cab changes. Uptown I was a prostitute, downtown a young mom. I did lots of commercials at the time—funny spots, like Lysol or taco commercials or anything where I had to be in a shower. Soon after getting my diagnosis, I walked into my agency and told them to take me off their rosters for a while. I needed to figure out if I was going to live past the next month, not whether I should wear the blue buttondown or the pink cap-sleeved shirt for the Tampax commercial. Once I stopped acting, my insurance dried up and it was COBRA time: More bucks for less bang. At least I didn't let it lapse.

"There is no end. There is no beginning. There is only the passion for life."
—FEDERICO FELLINI,
ITALIAN FILMMAKER

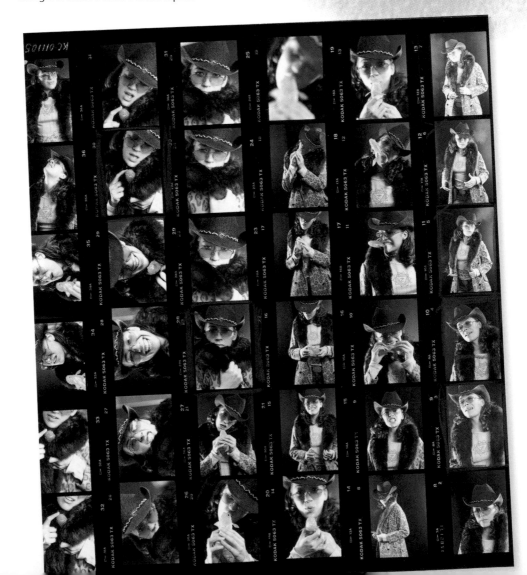

remember:

Take full advantage of your Cancer Card membership.
But use it, don't abuse it!

Swipe your card to get an out, or an in, for the aftermath of cancer
tantrums and for shopping therapy.

Beware the fine print: The Cancer Card doesn't get you out of taking
responsibility when you push too far or hurt someone.

Shopping boosts your immune system. No really, it does! So help
yourself to some retail therapy.

Bankruptcy, on the other hand, is not so therapeutic.

Be on the lookout for Cancer Card theft: Others can use your Cancer
Card against you.

Take heart: It is possible to keep working during your cancer fight.

Take heart: It is possible to not work during your cancer fight.

CHAPTER SIX 6

eat your veggies and SHAKE YOUR ASS

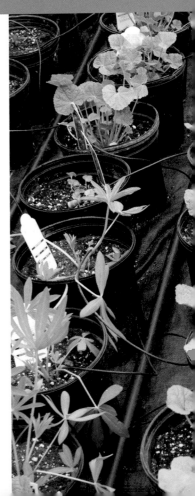

Remember the Milton Bradley game Operation? Well, before cancer forced me to educate myself, that juvenile game was my main reference for the body's organ systems. I was still looking for the "wishbone" when, out of nowhere, my vascular system blew up! Why hadn't I been paying attention? Why had I been strutting around in stupid acting classes? I should have gone to medical school; I should have listened in biology class instead of passing notes to my friends and flirting with pimply schoolboys. Oh, I wish I could go back and undo.

Get in line, right? Who doesn't feel that way about something? If only we could press STOP the moment before it all changed . . . but it just doesn't work that way. When the red phone rang with my wake-up call, a lightbulb went off.

Back then, I had no idea how to take care of myself, to eat right and nourish my body. My idea of nutrition was based on what to eat to keep (or whittle away) my figure for my job. PowerBars, coffee, fat-free this and take-out that: My meals were planned according to convenience. I didn't have time to cook! Order, pick up, or nuke, that pretty much describes my old routine. I chose restaurants based on wine lists, not the nutritional value of their food. Please, how square! The worst part about my ignorance was that I assumed it was my body's job to sort it all out. I put the junk in, and it dealt with it. I had no idea how, but that wasn't my problem. My job was to keep the junk on the table. Whatever my bod was doing, well, it just had to keep doing it, and if I drove my bus like a bat out of hell today, I promised I would slow it down tomorrow. I was in my twenties! Savings accounts, retirement packages, and fiber were for boring people! I wanted juicy, luscious living, and I didn't want to have to think about it. I was too cool for that.

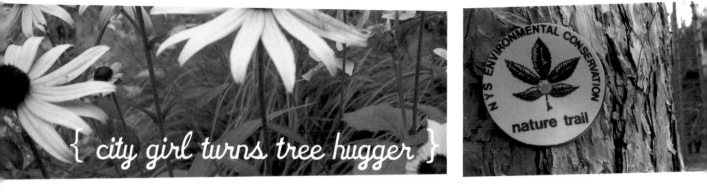

{ city girl turns tree hugger }

Then I got sick and my doctor said there was no cure. Holy shit! My damned body was asleep at the wheel. Or was I? Not that I thought I gave myself cancer, as some people wanted me to believe. Yet I couldn't help but wonder: In my ignorance, had I pulled the trigger on an already existing predisposition? Was my immune system struggling as I looked the other way, partied, and numbed out? I'll never know for sure, but it was certainly food for thought.

When my wonderful doctor told me to "watch and wait," I went nuts. *Hell no! I'm Stage IV—and there is no Stage V!* So I chose to explore alternative/holistic medicine, not because I wanted to be a brave pioneer, but because in my mind there were no other options. To watch and wait and do nothing felt totally disempowering. I wanted to be part of the solution, not part of the problem. So I gave it the ol' college try and read countless books on nutrition and natural recoveries from cancer. I traveled the country taking workshops and seminars, interviewing top researchers, Western doctors, Eastern doctors, teachers, gurus, alternative practitioners, nutritionists, naturopaths, yogis, and healers. I left no stone unturned and basically became a guinea pig with certifications. I did liver flushes, gallbladder cleanses, blood cleanses, I fasted, drank gallons of herbs (sock juice, as my dad calls the concoctions), downed supplements, and even drank my urine. (Once. Wine is much better.)

I spent a year driving back and forth to Philly to study at the Strengthening Health Institute (SHI), then went on to complete a health educator program at the Hippocrates Health Institute (HHI), a world-renowned healing center in Florida. It was there that the pieces of the puzzle finally began to fit together. The center teaches a living foods approach to healing through classes on cleansing and repairing the body with fresh, organic, uncooked and unrefined foods. It advocates a diet rich in enzymes and oxygen, both of which are essential for good health and are missing in the average American diet, which is high in meat, dairy, and refined processed foods.

Bringing my body back into balance was actually much simpler than I thought.

Here is the protocol I followed in a (wal)nut shell:

1. **Get back to nature** and back to the garden.

2. **Shake your booty.**

3. **Eat the right alkaline foods** that supply your body with oxygen and enzymes.

4. **Drink pure water.**

5. **Give your colon** a regular spring cleaning.

6. **Keep the stress level down** and the joy factor up.

7. **Snooze. Snooze. Snooze.**

If we create an environment where regeneration can occur, then "miracles"—actually the result of a commonsense approach to living and not so miraculous—can happen. It's that easy, but it also takes a colossal leap of faith and a willingness to break from the herd.

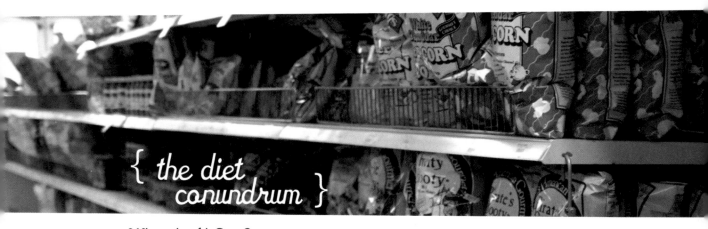

{ the diet conundrum }

What should I eat? Healthy or sick, it's a question that plagues us all. Low carbs? No carbs? Macrobiotics? South Beach? The Maker's Diet? The Blood Type Diet? It's so confusing, and it seems like everyone has the Holy Grail answer. Wouldn't it be great if we popped into this world with an owner's manual? *Hmm, I'm feeling a little short of breath; let me just go ahead and look that one up! Wow, I'm really constipated, turn to page 53!* Why doesn't one diet just take care of it all?

Instead of looking directly at the picture, look at the negative space around it. The one thing most reputable diets have in common isn't what they tell you to eat, it's what they tell you not to eat.

The body is phenomenally mysterious, and yet the answer to the diet conundrum is actually quite straightforward: "Eat food. Not too much. Mostly plants." I wish I could take credit for that one, but I can't. Michael Pollan came up with it in an article he wrote for the *New York Times Magazine*: "Unhappy Meals: 30 Years of Nutritional Science Has Made Americans Sicker, Fatter and Less Well Nourished. A Plea for the Return of Plain Old Food."

"But of course I eat food," you say. But do you? Food isn't made in a laboratory. Today we're infusing our food with tons of poisonous garbage not meant for human consumption! Chemicals, hormones, pesticides, and countless other toxic substances are clogging up and polluting both our inner and outer environments. Gardens are being replaced by test tubes, and the American public has become one big science experiment. The Standard American Diet, or SAD, is tap dancing on the last nerve of our health. In a world that runs on rapid globalization, SAD has spread like an aggressive cancer. As a result, the major health issues that are soaring in our country—diabetes, heart disease, obesity, and cancer—are now plaguing the entire planet. Thank you, Uncle Sam, for the globalization of illness. Bravo!

When we make the connection between what we consume and how we feel, a great transformational shift can occur. How many times do you select food for emotional comfort rather than fuel? Guess what the number one most consumed "vegetable" in this country is? The french fry. Number Two? Ketchup. Emotional comfort! Most people live to eat and don't eat to live. We scarf down our chow like we're hooked up to a feedbag and then wonder why we feel so bloated, cranky, and exhausted.

We wake up sick and tired on a daily basis. Allergies, high cholesterol, arthritis, lack of sex drive, low-level depression, and chronic diseases are just accepted parts of aging. We think it's normal to have a laundry list of aches and pains and feel depleted all the time. Well, it's not!

By the time you finish this chapter, you will be well on your way to creating your very own owner's manual.

If you find this information interesting and helpful, please continue educating yourself. I can only just scratch the surface here. Check out the appendix at the back of this book for loads of additional resources.

tip no.51

PUT THE LOVE
into your food

At first I found prepping and cooking my own food to be a real drag. But once I started to look at it as an expression of creativity and self-love, it began to take on sacred meaning. Now I read cookbooks like novels and geek out with highlighters and page tabs. My husband teases me about the pile on the nightstand, which threatens to topple over and bonk me on the head. One of my favorites is *The Raw Gourmet* by Nomi Shannon—very accessible and easy to understand. In it she writes: "Eating a high-enzyme diet consisting of raw fruit and vegetables, sprouted seeds, nuts, grains, and some seaweed will profoundly increase your chances of achieving optimal health. Eating predominately cooked food puts a tremendous strain on the body. The SAD diet of meat, bread, dairy, processed and cooked foods, caffeine and alcohol is not only totally enzymeless, it also creates an acid state in the body which causes a variety of health problems." To understand this concept, it's important to know what an enzyme is and how the pH of the body can affect your overall health.

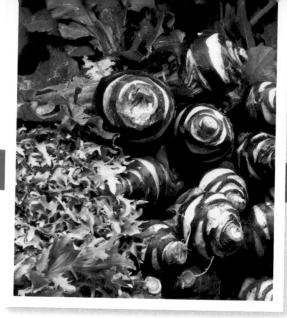

tip no.**52**

ADD SOME ENZYME
enlightenment

Enzymes are little protein catalysts that create complex chemical reactions in the cells of every living plant and animal. Everything from blinking, food digestion, and DNA repair happens as a result of the enzyme dynamos busy at work. Even our immune system relies on enzymes to attack and kill viruses, bacteria, and pesky cancer cells. Dr. Edward Howell, enzyme pioneer, describes enzymes as the substances that make all life possible: "Without enzymes, no activity at all would take place. Neither vitamins, minerals, nor hormones can do any work—without enzymes. Think of it this way: Enzymes are the 'labor force' that build your body just like construction workers are the labor force that build your house. You may have all the necessary building materials and lumber, but to build a house you need workers, which represent the vital life element." Through Howell's discoveries, the first digestive enzyme supplements were created. Today they are the cornerstone of my supplement regime; I take them with every meal (especially cooked meals) and as a result see a real difference in my overall energy and digestive function.

Unfortunately, we are born with limited enzymatic reserves. Big bummer! Here's another image for you: Your body is a bank account, and enzymes are the currency. Imagine making deposits instead of constant withdrawals. The more deposits you make, the better your metabolism and immune system work. By eating a mostly raw vegetarian diet—which is loaded with its own enzymes—you can increase your reserves and have much more energy. On the other hand, cooking food above 118 degrees (as well as the pasteurization process) destroys enzymes and inevitably leads to energy bankruptcy. Processed foods are also devoid of enzymes. So when we eat these foods, our body is forced to pull enzymes from other areas, including our muscles, glands, and organs, to aid in the digestion process. In essence, our bodies rebuild the food so that it resembles its original enzymatic form; then we can digest and absorb it. What a waste of time and energy! Raw and living foods—those that are still growing, like sprouts—contain their own enzymes. We don't have to steal from our own reserves to digest them. They come to the party with everything they need and don't drain the host!

OXYGEN AND A HEALTHY pH BALANCE
are cancer's worst enemies

Let's turn to another key player on Team Survival. What do you need most to live? Oxygen! In 1931 scientist Otto Warburg won a Nobel Prize for the connection he discovered between oxygen and cancer. His studies showed that the number one cause of cancer is a lack of oxygen in the cellular environment. Warburg determined that cancer cells are anaerobic, which means they thrive in an oxygen-depleted environment. Conversely, they cannot live in an oxygen-rich environment. Are you starting to catch on?

You need to design a diet high in oxygen to choke out the cancer cells and take back the night!

When a body is too acidic and living in an anaerobic state, the stage is set for a host of ailments ranging from chronic fatigue to degenerative disease.

If you spaced out in science class like I did, you might not remember that the pH scale goes from 0 to 14, with 7 being neutral. Below 7 is acid; above 7, alkaline. The optimal blood pH level is 7.365. You can check your urine pH level with pH strips. It's easy: Just pee on a little piece of litmus paper and measure the reading. The lower the number, the more acidic you are.

In his book *The pH Miracle*, my friend Dr. Robert Young uses a simple image to get the message across: "Think of your body as a fish tank," he writes. "Imagine your cells and organ systems as fish, bathed in fluids (including the blood) that transport food and remove wastes. Then suppose I back up a car and put the tailpipe up against the air intake filter that supplies oxygen to the tank. The water becomes filled with carbon dioxide making it too acidic. Then I throw in too much food, or the wrong kind of food, and the fish are unable to consume or digest it all, so it starts to decompose. How long before the fish are goners?"

An acidic environment makes us sick—just like the fish. On the other hand, an alkaline environment floods our bodies with oxygen, keeping us vibrant and healthy. No matter how zapped I am, when I drink fresh veggie juice (hugely alkalizing) I feel like a wilted plant come back to life. How can we change the environment our cells swim in to keep them clean and nourished?

The best way to increase the alkalinity of our bodies is to adopt a vegetarian diet with a high concentration of raw foods.

I can just hear the outcry this suggestion will cause: "Wait, stop right there! Are you asking me to become a vegetarian—or worse, a liberal?! No way! First of all, I don't want to live like a rabbit, and second, how am I supposed to resist those intoxicating aromas bubbling from the stove?" Well, suck in those aromas because that's where the majority of the vitamins and minerals are going: into the air. If you're not ready for a wholesale change to your eating habits, then just adopt as many (or as few) of my recommendations as you want. Even a small change will make a difference. As for living like a bunny, think Playboy or Energizer Bunny, because raw and living foods not only help repair and heal the body, but give you tons of energy and make you hot as well!

A 100 percent raw diet is optimum. But most people do well with an 80/20 raw diet, which means 80 percent of your plate is covered with salads or raw cuisine and 20 percent with cooked foods, like a side dish.

Check out the resources section at the back of this book for a list of my favorite cookbooks and Web sites, along with a few great recipes. Why not give it a try? Consider it a little experiment. You'll be surprised at how amazing you feel and what a huge selection of delicious raw and living foods recipes there are to choose from. I promise you won't just be nibbling on lettuce. No way! Life is meant to be sweet and savory, bitter and sour, and you deserve to enjoy every morsel of it. But to do that, you must educate yourself on the power of the food choices we make.

tip no.54

PLEASE PASS THE *chlorophyll*

At the top of the list of those food choices should be chlorophyll. Think about it: Chlorophyll is the substance in plants that allows them to absorb light from the sun and convert that light into usable energy. Our very existence depends on the sun. We are interconnected to its energy on many levels, including what we shove in our mouths. Life is a tender exchange, a circle of giving and receiving. Plants take in carbon dioxide and give off oxygen; we take in oxygen and give off carbon dioxide; everybody's happy, end of story.

Here's some cool geek trivia: Chlorophyll is chemically related to blood. The difference is that the main atom in hemoglobin (blood's oxygen transporter) is iron, while in chlorophyll it's magnesium. Chlorophyll contains a powerful blood builder that's said to increase red blood cells, improve circulation, ease inflammation, oxygenate the body, and counteract harmful free radicals. By eating a diet high in chlorophyll (raw fruits and veggies, especially leafy greens), we dine on liquid oxygen, the very substance we need to stay alive and thrive.

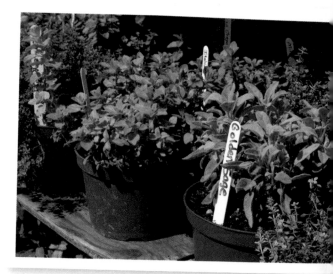

LEARN THE
raw facts

We are electric currents, and so is our food. Nutrient-depleted foods leave our bodies still feeling hungry. So what do we do? We eat more crap. When you think of malnourished people, you probably picture emaciated famine victims. In fact many average-weight to over-weight people are malnourished, thanks to the poor quality of the food they consume and the condition of their colons.

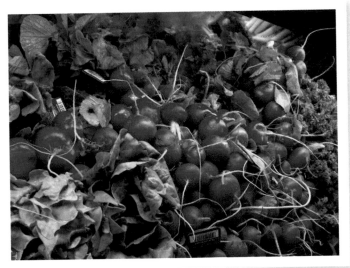

Dr. Brian Clement, one of my teachers and a director of HHI, clearly explains what happens to cooked and processed foods and how they affect our bodies: "During this apparently harmless process vital enzymes are destroyed, proteins are coagulated (making them very difficult to assimilate), vitamins are mostly destroyed with the remainder changing into forms that are difficult for the body to utilize. Pesticides are restructured into even more toxic compounds, valuable oxygen is lost, and free radicals are produced. Studies suggest that cooked proteins are up to 50% less likely to be utilized. Oxygen, enzymes, phytonutrients and hormones are consequently destroyed. In addition. . . . cooking food above a certain temperature (slightly under 200 degrees Fahrenheit) causes a pathogenic response in the body called leukocytosis, whereby white blood cells are used to digest food much as they would attack a foreign substance."

Generally a jump in white blood cells is the body's response to infection. Even foods that aren't cooked but are high in refined sugars, carbs, preservatives, and chemicals raise your leukocites (white blood cell count). Dr. Paul Kouchakoff was the first scientist to discover that food eaten raw does not produce the same effects as cooked food. In fact, if we keep our cooked food intake to 20 to 30 percent of our diet with the remainder of our plates filled with fresh veggies, we can offset leukocytosis. Wow, doesn't that just make you wanna grab a salad? I don't know about you, but I want my immune system to focus on taking out cancer cells, not Tater Tots and Twinkies!

TAKE OUT *the trash*

No matter how healthy our diets, if our inner sewer system is clogged our bodies break down. We need a clean and healthy colon to absorb the nutrients from the food we eat and to eliminate waste and toxins. Most, if not all, of us have impacted and encrusted colons from years of eating meat, dairy, processed foods, breads, candies, cookies, bad oils, and other tasty (but toxic) treats.

Did you know that the average person is hauling around between seven and ten extra pounds just in the colon? As a matter of fact, medical examiners have noted up to fifty or sixty pounds of impacted fecal matter during routine autopsies. "How is that possible?" you ask. Well, the intestines are twenty-six feet long, and if you were to spread them out, their surface—including all the nooks, crannies and intestinal villi—would cover a tennis court. Get the picture? Basically when the pipes get backed up, the stagnant food rots and hardens, causing myriad problems, including lack of absorption of the good stuff food has to offer and low production of good bacteria. How can someone be obese and malnourished at the same time? Lining the walls of the small intestine are lots of the aforementioned little hairy guys called villi. When food passes over them, they draw in nutrients. But if they're encrusted with fecal matter, the nutrients just zoom on by. Or they sit there unabsorbed and get stinky.

Like everything in life, it's all about balance. Good bacteria and bad bacteria share space in our colons. But if we compromise the terrain through our food choices, the bad guys take over.

These little undertakers push the inner compost button, decomposing our bodies while we're still inhabiting them. I don't know about you, but I really don't want to be decomposing while I'm naively walking around in my UGGs and complaining that skinny jeans are back in style.

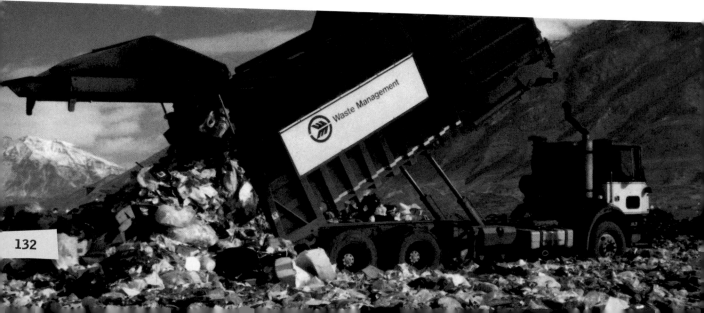

Some experts believe that if you aren't moving your bowels three times a day, you should consider yourself constipated. There may be days', even weeks' worth of debris (especially if you eat animal products) just hanging out and clogging you up. The sad thing is that most of us barely have one bowel movement per day. In his book *The Cure: Heal Your Body, Save Your Life*, Dr. Timothy Brantley adds up a staggering constipation calculation: "If you are only having three bowel movements per week and the norm is three bowel movements PER DAY, by the end of the week you will be 18 bowel movements short. After a month, you will be short 72 bowel movements, at the end of the year you will be short 864 bowel movements and over an 80 year lifespan, you will be short 70,000 bowel movements!" Gross!

Once we begin the cleansing process, even more trash is dumped into the colon and bloodstream, so it's important to keep moving the waste—move it out!

how to
UNCLOG YOUR PIPES

Okay, don't freak out and get squirmy or prudish. But the best way to take out the trash is through an internal bath: an enema or colonic. Enemas are a great way to get the lower bowels moving and grooving. Enemas are a snap. Just follow the directions on the box, deck out your bathroom detox ashram, and go to town. Colonics are even better because they access the ascending, transverse, and descending intestines. An average session lasts from forty-five minutes to an hour. In the beginning it's best to do a series; the number of treatments you'll need really depends on the condition of your colon.

Some people who oppose colon therapy claim that it's unnatural, and that you can become dependent on it. The concern is that folks will overdo it, going too frequently. Another criticism is that it washes away good bacteria. First of all, it's unnatural to be living in such a highly toxic time; we need to think outside the box, especially when we have something as unnatural as cancer to contend with. Next, colon therapy will not make you dependent. Think of it like a workout: The gentle pressure from the water actually tones and rebuilds your muscles by making peristalsis—the contraction of smooth muscles that propels stuff through the digestive tract—stronger. Once the initial cleansing process is complete, colonics need only be used for maintenance and upkeep. Lastly, good bacteria can only breed in a clean environment. A probiotic can be taken after cleansing to help repopulate the colon with good bacteria. Eventually the colon will rebalance itself, especially when all the debris is cleared away. Until the invention of laxatives (which only exacerbate the situation and are sometimes harmful—they can cause dehydration, among other problems), enemas were widely used by our grandparents and accepted by local doctors. In fact, they have long been considered one of the best remedies for a headache!

To find a good colonics practitioner, flip to the resources section at the back of the book or ask a local chiropractor or naturopath to recommend someone. Remember, we're not only what we eat but also what we don't poop!

tip no.57

ORDER A
wheatgrass chaser

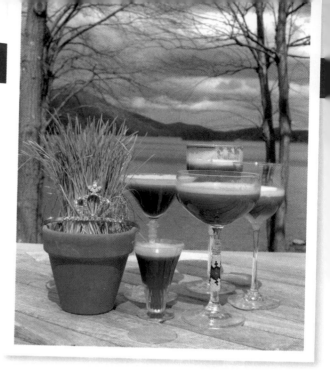

Wheatgrass can be a powerful tonic for healing through both internal consumption and rectal implantation. One four-ounce shot is like hooking your immune system up to a set of jumper cables. Those magic mini lawns are filled with liquid sunshine. Some of the benefits of regular consumption of wheatgrass juice include better circulation, a stronger immune system, fewer free radicals, and increased energy. On top of that, wheatgrass is an excellent source of vitamins A, C, and E, most of the B vitamins, and a compound called laetrile, which some believe to have anti-tumor properties. Wheatgrass also has tons of minerals and is a great source of protein. Check your local health food store or grow your own. To enjoy wheatgrass at home, you'll need a special juicer to pull the juice out of the grass, but you don't have to get fancy. Mine is a little hand-crank plastic job that I got for $28—great for travel and easy to clean.

SOMETHING TO CHEW ON

Chewing can help with constipation. Digestion begins in your mouth. In fact, nutrition experts say you should drink your food and chew your water, which basically means that everything that goes down your throat should be pureed, because digestion starts in your mouth. So start grinding those purdy jaws!

Not only does the nectar of this lovely green blade make for a fortifying beverage, but it's also a great lower bowel emptier. Wheatgrass implants stimulate peristalsis and replenish the electrolytes in your colon.

Colon hydrotherapy with a wheatgrass chaser is a good deal for the big daddy of all organs, too—your liver. Once implanted, a portion of the juice travels through the hepatic vein directly to the liver, stimulating it to purge and cleanse and giving it a great boost of the mighty healer chlorophyll (think oxygen). Your liver is the chief organ of elimination. Think of it as the body's recycling center, constantly filtering and cleaning the blood. The liver also plays a strong role in digestion, assimilation, your immune system, and literally hundreds of other processes. It's one busy dude! Once it gets clogged, so do you.

BECOME A
food matchmaker

Another way to help with digestion and assimilation is proper food combining. Different foods require different digestive enzymes. In addition, different foods have different transit schedules. When we combine food properly, the traffic in our gut moves easily. When we don't, however, digestive enzymes are neutralized—and the resulting traffic jam fouls up our digestion. In *The Raw Food Detox Diet*, author Natalia Rose refers to food combining as "quick exit combinations." As Rose says, "The quicker the food is digested the less waste matter it will leave." Remember, if you're eating food

that takes a long time to be broken down, then your energy is being consumed by digestion rather than renewal. Here's just one example from Rose's book: An avocado and toast takes three to four hours to digest, while an egg and toast takes about eight hours (in the stomach alone) to digest. Think about what happens when you eat regular meals that are poorly combined. Eventually there's sure to be a pileup!

While some people can be more lenient, my system tends to be pretty straightforward. You can tell if a combination works for you by the amount of bloating or gas you feel after the meal.

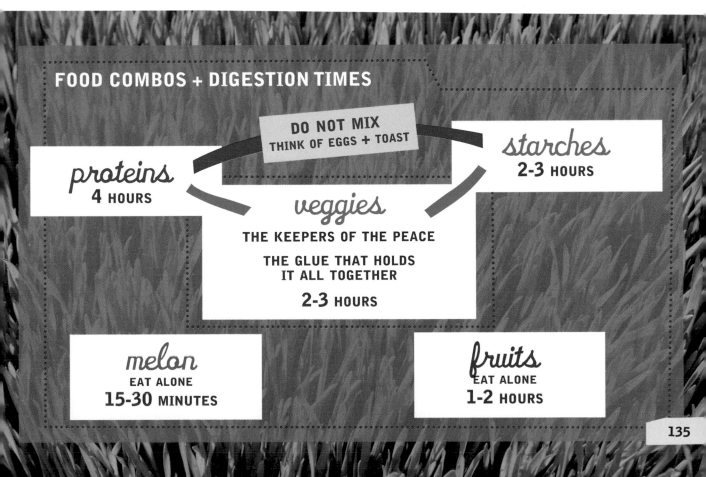

FOOD COMBOS + DIGESTION TIMES

DO NOT MIX
THINK OF EGGS + TOAST

proteins
4 HOURS

starches
2-3 HOURS

veggies
THE KEEPERS OF THE PEACE

**THE GLUE THAT HOLDS
IT ALL TOGETHER**

2-3 HOURS

melon
EAT ALONE
15-30 MINUTES

fruits
EAT ALONE
1-2 HOURS

SORRY, FELLOW WINOS!

Another tip to remember is to try not to consume liquids while eating. They dilute the digestive juices.

tip no.59

DRINK PURE WATER—
lots of it!

I cannot overemphasize the importance of drinking good water. Like the earth, we are made up of 70 percent water and 30 percent mass. Water is not coffee, tea, soda, bottled juice, pasteurized dairy, or so-called energy drinks. Water is essential for every bodily function, including my favorite topic, elimination. Without proper hydration, our cells, tissues, and organs wither on the vine. For staying hydrated at home, it's best to get a water filtration device—tap water is loaded with chemicals (like chlorine, which wipes out bacteria in the colon) and heavy metals. Remember, if you don't filter your water, your body will. Bottled waters are better, though plastic containers aren't so great, but we can't always be perfect. One thing I do advise if you're drinking bottled water is to check the pH of the brand. If you're really industrious, you can find charts on the Internet that will provide you with that information. Believe it or not, many waters are highly acidic. Trinity is a good brand to choose, with a pH of more than 9.

Distilled water is an excellent choice.

Distilled water is totally pure (but devoid of minerals). You can boost its alkalinity with pH drops (which reoxygenate). Distilled water can also be remineralized by adding a pinch of Celtic Sea Salt or Himalayan sea salt. (These are the only salts you should be using; table salt is bleached, refined, highly cooked, and stripped of minerals.)

Another option is Penta water, which is specially processed to feature smaller molecules than regular water. This means it penetrates the cells better.

Check this out: We need to drink between 50 and 75 percent of our body weight in ounces each day! Dr. Young suggests that while we're healing, we need to drink a liter for every thirty pounds. So if you weigh 120 pounds, you should drink four liters of water throughout the course of your day. Though I try, I never quite get that much down. Do what you can and start guzzling!

SOME NOTES ON GRAINS AND PASTA

- Choose whole grains like spelt and Kamut. If it's white, it's processed! Geeky fact: One grain of white rice in a cup of water will rot. One grain of brown rice in a cup of water will sprout.

- I use soba noodles a lot for pasta because they're really easy to digest. Try to keep them al dente, or they get really mushy.

- If you have a problem with wheat allergies—aka celiac disease, which can really do a number on your digestion—switch to gluten-free grains like buckwheat, brown rice, flaxseed, millet, and quinoa.

- Did you know you can eat pasta raw? You'll need to buy a spiralizer (about $25 online), which allows you to make groovy noodles out of veggies like squash, zucchini, and even pumpkin. No matter what you choose, though, try to stay 70/30 or 80/20!

{ where's the protein and calcium? }

If you're with me so far and have decided to dip your toe into this way of life, you may be thinking, *Okay, so now I'm eating lots of veggies and detoxing my body—great. But what about protein and calcium? Where do I get those?* This is probably the main question that every vegetarian is asked. These fears stem from a lack of education and false messages sent out by advertisers. We are conditioned to believe that if we don't get enough milk and steak (because people think those are the only real sources of calcium and protein—gimme a break!), we'll turn into little weaklings who shrivel up and die. Wrong! The truth is that we can get all the protein we need from plant-based foods. Did you know that fruits, leafy greens, veggies, sprouts, wheatgrass, chlorella (a single-celled green alga), blue-green algae, and hemp seeds, to name just a few, kick burger ass? Dark leafy greens in particular are a terrific source of protein; they're also very high in iron and calcium. Broccoli, sesame seeds, almonds, and seaweed are other fantastic (and absorbable) sources of calcium. In fact, studies by the American Heart Association have shown that vegetarians absorb and retain more calcium from foods than non-vegetarians.

{ got mucus? }

One of the main problems with a diet heavy in animal products is that it's incredibly acidic. Acidic foods create mucus in the body, and mucus acts like glue, clogging our elimination organs. Also, remember that acidity lowers the pH of the body, creating an environment for cancer cells to thrive in. Many nutrition experts believe that humans are ill equipped to fully digest and absorb meat. Consider a true carnivore, the lovely lioness. She has fangs to tear, a short and sweet digestive tract, and an abundance of hydrochloric acid to do the tough job of digesting flesh. Zebra goes in, zebra comes out. Now think of what you've learned about the length of our intestines. Pig goes in; pig stays in for days and weeks at a time, corrupts the internal environment, and creates stagnation that bad bacteria (remember those little undertakers?) just adore. Oh, and don't forget about leukocytosis! All in all, if you really want to see your white blood cell count skyrocket (in a bad way), eat some animal products. Your immune system will deploy the troops big-time.

Here's another fact: Cooked meat increases the risk of developing . . . what else? You guessed it, cancer! Gold star. Even the National Cancer Institute and the American Institute for Cancer Research (AICR) verify that little gem. The more well-done the meat, the more carcinogenic it becomes. The carcinogens damage your DNA by emitting dangerous radioactivity. Frying, broiling, and barbecuing meat are to be especially avoided due to the high temperatures used in these methods. One AICR study found that people who ate the most red meat (more than 2.8 ounces a day) had a 17 percent greater risk of colon cancer than those who ate the least. The same amount of processed red meats (hot dogs, lunch meat, and so on) caused an even greater increase in risk. Red meat can also damage the DNA of colon cells and increase the formation of certain cancer-causing compounds within the gut. This supports the need to cleanse and either cut way back on or, ideally, eliminate these products. Aflatoxins are also carcinogenic. These are fungi that can be found in peanuts, peanut butter, and stored grains, but also in the milk of animals given contaminated feed.

Dr. T. Colin Campbell, professor emeritus of nutritional biochemistry at Cornell University, is a brilliant researcher who pioneered the investigation of the diet–cancer link in his writings, including *The China Study: The Most Comprehensive Study of Nutrition Ever Conducted and the Startling Implications for Diet, Weight Loss and Long-Term Health*. Place this book on your must-read list today! It clears up the fallacies of our modern diet and provides some thought-provoking answers to the question *What really causes cancer?* One of the biggest contenders: a diet that is higher than 10 percent animal protein! Americans eat way more than that. Dr. Campbell found that the protein that consistently creates cancer is casein, which makes up 87 percent of the protein in cow's milk. He estimates that "80% to 90%

of all cancers, cardiovascular diseases, and other degenerative illness can be prevented, at least until very old age, simply by adopting a plant-based diet."

{ *milk: it does the body bad* }

We have been led to believe that milk is an essential part of good health. In reality, dairy milk contributes to the overall breakdown of our systems. Drinking too much of it can actually contribute to calcium depletion in our bodies. Here's how: Calcium is mostly stored in our bones and teeth. As I've noted, a high-protein animal-based diet is extremely acidic. Calcium is an alkaline mineral. Therefore, our bodies mine calcium from our bones to neutralize the acids created by the glass of milk we just downed. So it turns out that milk has the opposite effect of what we've been led to believe. If you really want strong bones, pasteurized milk shouldn't be your main source of calcium.

Milk is also one of the most common causes of food allergies. We simply don't have the enzyme needed to digest it. A cow drinks cow's milk. A bunny drinks bunny's milk. Do you ever see them switch and swap?

TITILLATING FACTS FROM *THE CHINA STUDY* BY DR. COLIN CAMPBELL

- Populations that consume more animal protein have higher blood cholesterol levels, which in turn are linked to greater rates of heart disease and cancer.
- Experimental animal research has consistently shown that proteins from animal sources promote higher cholesterol levels than proteins from plant sources.
- A high-animal-protein diet allows more dangerous chemical carcinogens into our cells and facilitates the process by which these carcinogens are transformed by enzymes then bound to our DNA, creating cancer. In experiments, plant protein has been shown to inhibit these processes.
- Animal protein has been found to promote high levels of insulin-like growth factor I, or IGF-1, which in turn has been found to be a predictor of certain cancers.
- Women consuming diets high in animal-based protein produce greater amounts of reproductive hormones, which are linked to higher rates of breast cancer.
- Diets high in animal protein have been shown to exacerbate the formation of kidney stones and draw calcium out of the bones, encouraging osteoporosis.
- Conversely, diets that derive most of their protein from a rich variety of unrefined vegetables, legumes, and whole grains have the ability to prevent and sometimes even treat the conditions mentioned above, including heart disease, certain cancers, kidney stones, and osteoporosis.

MAKE SMARTER
milk and meat choices

If you really can't see yourself giving up milk and meat, at least choose the best quality. Raw foodies advocate the use of raw (unpasteurized) goat's milk as an alternative to cow's milk because it's much easier to digest and is closer to the consistency of human milk. You can wean yourself off of cow's milk with rice, oat, almond, or soy milks (in moderation) as well. Also, meat should be organic, grass fed, and consumed in small portions. Picture it as a side dish next to loads of veggies and a big salad. The American Dietetic Association came up with a good visual: The average serving of meat, it says, should be the size of a deck of cards.

This information can be tough to swallow for folks who were raised on animal products. It certainly was for me. I grew up across the street from a dairy farm! I'll never forget auditioning for the movie *Annie* when I was a kid. Though I didn't get the role (I totally choked), I did receive a year's supply of Ovaltine! Perfect for my afternoon shake. And there was no shortage of meat around, either. My grandmother was a chef who grabbed every chance she got to cook up a hunk of flesh. Tongue-and-Spam sandwiches were a favorite in our house. Looking back, I can see why becoming a veggie-head was easy for me! Of course we all have different constitutions—Grandma lived to ninety-three. Granted, she suffered from debilitating arthritis, diverticulitis, and high cholesterol for the last thirty years of her life, but she didn't have cancer! Remember, though, the products available today are not the same as what our grandparents ate back in the day.

Agribusiness relies on quantity, speed, and the increasing demands for cheaper products. As a result, the animals now raised for our consumption are jacked up with hormones, antibiotics, herbicides, pesticides, and other medications that ultimately find their way into our rivers, land, and bloodstreams.

CHECK INTO
fat rehab

You know it's true. Every woman I know needs rehabilitation when it comes to her stance on fat. We're all so brainwashed by the low-fat, fat-free craze that we've damaged our ability to make proper judgments. "A moment on the lips, a lifetime on the hips." How many of us have that saying branded on the brain? Ever find yourself on a fat-free pig-out binge from hell? Why not eat the whole box of cookies, they're fat-free! Pass the fat-free ice cream! If you'd just given your body something lusciously rich (and healthy), your wild woman cravings would have been satisfied. Rather than teeter on the verge of coming undone, give your body what it needs.

"Good fats" are necessary for proper brain function, a strong immune system, hormone production, strengthening cell walls, joint lubrication, organ protection, and a healthy nervous system.

They are also clean and sustainable sources of energy. Good fats help us absorb and transport vitamins and, believe it or not, actually help us detox, increase metabolism, lose weight, and lessen the appearance of cellulite. Hallelujah! Bad fats (saturated and partially hydrogenated or trans fats) are the hip and health busters. Run, don't walk away from those.

So what are good fats? Unsaturated fats, the king of which are essential fatty acids. EFAs are often classified in two groups: omega-3s and omega-6s. They are where it's at! EFAs get their name from the fact that they are essential (duh!) and cannot be produced in your body; you have to get them from your grub. Great sources of EFAs are cold-pressed extra-virgin olive oil, avocados, kiwi, lingonberries, purslane greens, nuts, seeds (including hemp, pumpkin, and especially flaxseeds), and fatty fish.

Though technically a saturated fat, coconut oil is terrific for you, too. It generally gets a bad rap because of the partially hydrogenated kind, but in its natural and unrefined form coconut is healing and delicious. Coconuts contain lauric acid, the same wonderful substance that is found in breast milk and that boosts immunity. Look for young Thai coconuts, whose meat is loaded with good fats and

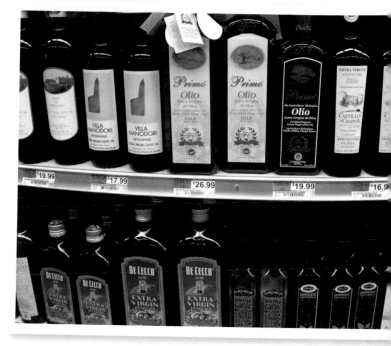

nutrients. Coconut water is also a fantastic source of electrolytes, and coconuts boost metabolism and have anti-viral and anti-fungal properties. Add them to your smoothies and look out, world! Geeky fact: Coconut water is nearly identical to our blood plasma. In fact, it was used in World War II for emergency blood transfusions. Cool!

In general, raw fats are much better for you and your liver than cooked fats and oils. When cooking with oils, stick with coconut (the very best for high heat), olive, and sesame, which can all handle higher heats. Lightly sautéing is key, or pouring the oil on afterward. Other oils that are great for salads (though they're too delicate for cooking) include flax, hemp, Udo's Choice (a brand of blended oils), macadamia nut, and walnut. Stay away from margarine and shortening (aka trans fats), commercial cooking sprays, vegetable, corn, and peanut oil. They wreak havoc. It's also best to avoid butter, but if you just gotta have it, look for raw organic versions.

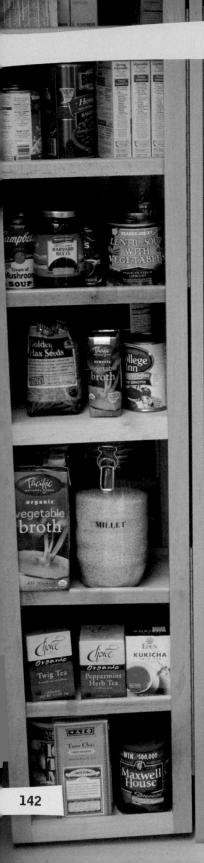
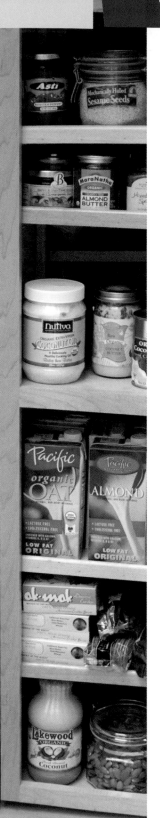

DO AN ALL-OUT
pantry raid!

Time for immune system boot camp! Now more than ever you need to assist your body. Think of it as your sacred space, a living altar. Consistently care for and revere it every single day. Try it and see how you feel. Once you get over the detox hump, you will more than likely experience a sense of vitality like you've never felt before. Start by cleaning out your pantry.

- **Out with all things white** and processed.

- **Read the labels.** If you can't pronounce it, your body can't digest it.

- **If it has a shelf life longer** than a human's life expectancy, it's sure to shorten your shelf life.

- **Adios to hydrogenated oils** and cooked animal fats, artificial colors, flavors, fat-free crap, fake food, and sodas.

- **Try to avoid all refined sugar** and cut back on fruit while you're dealing with the big C. Many alternative practitioners believe that sugar not only suppresses the immune system, but also feeds the cancer cells! How so? Well diets high in sugar cause blood sugar levels to spike. Once that happens the body releases a hormone called insulin to bring blood sugar levels back to normal. One of insulin's many functions is to promote cell growth, whether we're talking normal cells or cancer cells. So the more sugar you eat, the more insulin is circulating in the body and thus the more opportunity for cancer cells to grow and divide—need I say more?

{let's go shopping}

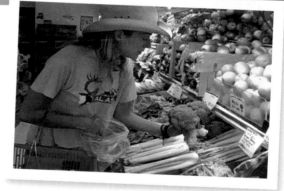

An empty pantry is a recipe for bad food choices. Think of your pantry as an arsenal: Keeping it properly stocked will help you win the healthy eating battle. Grocery shopping can be a ritual, a way to honor your body.

The best way to shop in a supermarket or health food store is to focus your attention on the periphery. That's where the fresh food is.

The middle aisles are usually where you can get yourself into trouble. Those aisles tend to be a crack den of sugar and processed food central.

CRAZY SEXY SHOPPING LIST

Here's a short list of foods you'll find in my personal cache. Some are healing staples, while others are transitional foods. All are a diet upgrade.

- *Grains and noodles.* Millet, quinoa, buckwheat, spelt, and Kamut grains or pastas and soba noodles.
- *Raw nuts and seeds.* Always buy fresh raw nuts; roasted nuts are rancid. Almonds, pecans, walnuts, macadamia nuts, hazelnuts, pine nuts, pumpkin seeds, flaxseeds (either buy a small grinder for these or buy them already ground), sesame seeds, hemp seeds, and sunflower seeds. Also raw almond butter and tahini—it's like peanut butter, only made with sesame seeds. Yum! Note: Soaking nuts makes them more digestible; it removes the enzyme inhibitors that keep them from spoiling.

- *Seaweed.* Nori, dulse, arame, hijiki.
- *Veggies, veggies, and more veggies.* Cucumbers, broccoli, kale, celery, parsley, cabbage, romaine and green lettuce, spinach, peppers, zucchini, asparagus, chard, green beans, alfalfa sprouts, lentil sprouts, mung bean sprouts, sweet pea and sunflower sprouts, onions, garlic, leeks, cauliflower, fresh herbs, eggplant, winter squash, carrots, arugula, bok choy, sweet potatoes . . . the list is endless! Note: Storing your veggies in bags will help them last longer.
- *Fruits.* Avocados and tomatoes (yes, they are technically fruits), apples, lemons, limes, grapefruit, watermelon, pears, grapes, and berries. Low-glycemic fruits (those that are less sweet, like blueberries) are generally better than high-glycemic fruits (such as bananas) while you're healing. Remember to consume fruit in moderation, if at all.
- *Breads.* Sprouted breads are the best, because they have more nutrients and are much easier to digest. My favorite brands are Ezekiel and Manna. For tortillas (great for wraps), I like Alvarado Street Sprouted Wheat. Ezekiel also makes cereals—try them with rice or oat milk. You can also use almond milk, though it's not a great food combo.
- *Sweetener.* Stevia, a powerful herb with no sugar, comes in packets. Let me tell you, a little goes a long way. A small amount of agave can also be used, although it's very sweet.
- *Oils for salad dressing.* Udo's Choice oil blends, flaxseed oil, cold-pressed olive oil, macadamia nut oil, walnut oil, hemp seed oil.
- *Oils for light cooking.* Coconut oil (the most stable of all oils) and cold-pressed olive oil. It's best to buy oils packaged in dark bottles and to store them in a cool dark place.
- *Seasonings.* Get creative and experiment with different herbs. Fresh and organic is better, but if you can't get fresh, at least buy organic. Use Celtic or Himalayan sea salt, Nama Shoyu, Bragg's Liquid Aminos, and miso.
- *Other good snacks and quick foods.* Spelt or brown rice cakes, Ryvita crackers, Lydia's raw crackers and cereals, fresh salsa (made with lemon or lime juice, not vinegar), hummus, oil-cured olives, tempeh, SoyBoy raviolis, veggie burgers, veggie meatballs, Amy's organic products, air-popped popcorn, Guiltless Gourmet chips, sweet potato chips, and LaraBars (great for travel).
- *Appliances.* A juicer, Cuisinart, salad spinner, and blender are the main appliances you'll need to get started. Oh, and a good knife!
- *Remember to read labels.* Watch for acidic ingredients such as yeast, citric acid, vinegar, peanuts, and corn syrup.

{ brenda cobb's story }

As you've probably already guessed,

I am passionate about nutrition. Getting to
where I am today with my healthy eating
principles and beliefs has been quite a journey.
As with everything else on my Crazy Sexy
Cancer quest, I left no stone unturned. I met
many helpful and inspiring folks along the way.
One of my most trusted mentors and teachers
is an amazing woman named Brenda Cobb. I
met Brenda during a lecture she was giving
at a health expo in New York, and we hit it off
immediately. Brenda helped me realize that
eating healthy isn't just something you do at
home; it's something you can apply when you're
out at restaurants—even corner diners! When
I first met her, she took me to a local diner and
showed me how to make healthy menu choices.
Now I apply those healthy ordering skills anytime I eat out. Below Brenda tells the story of
her own journey:

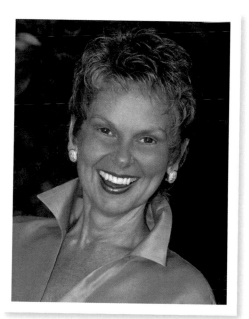

Nutrition expert Brenda Cobb

Brenda:

In February 1999 I was diagnosed with
breast and cervical cancer. My doctor
told me that if I didn't have surgery,
chemotherapy, and radiation, I would be
dead in six months to a year. I chose not
to follow the doctor's recommendations
because I had family members who had
had cervical, breast, uterine, and ovarian cancers; they did surgery, chemo,
and radiation, and their cancers came
back with a vengeance—or they died
from the treatments. I wanted to find a
natural way to help my body heal. I discovered raw and living foods, and it just
made sense to me that if I cleansed and
detoxed my body and took in optimum
nutrition, my body would heal itself.

And that's exactly what happened.
In six months I was cancer-free. I knew

that I had to share this information with others, so I opened the Living Foods Institute and began teaching others my healthy lifestyle principles. Even my doctor began to send his patients to my center. I've helped thousands of people with cancer and all types of diseases to heal naturally. I have come to realize that it's never too late and there are no hopeless, incurable, terminal diseases when people are willing to change their way of thinking, heal the emotional stuff buried deep inside, eat organic raw and living foods, and cleanse the blood and the colon. The body is amazing and can be healed of almost anything. Time and again I have witnessed people completely healing when no one thought it was possible.

On the day I was diagnosed, I thought it was the most horrible day of my life, but now I realize that it was the best blessing I have ever received. It truly changed my life and my direction. Through this seemingly difficult situation, I discovered my mission and purpose in life: to help others to find their own natural way of healing.

"My only regret in life is that I did not drink more champagne."
—JOHN MAYNARD KEYNES, ECONOMIST

THE CRAZY, SEXY HEALING DIET: AN OVERVIEW

Here's a quick roundup of the diet that both Brenda Cobb and I advocate:

- *Eat vegan only!* No animal or dairy products of any kind, cooked or raw. Animal and dairy products are acidic. They create mucus and cause digestion, assimilation, and elimination problems. Meat rots and putrefies in the body and gives off uric acid. You want an alkaline body!

- *Eat organic food.* Chemicals on and in conventional produce are toxic. Chemical toxicity is one of the major reasons people get sick. If a pesticide can kill bugs, just imagine what it must be doing to your insides!

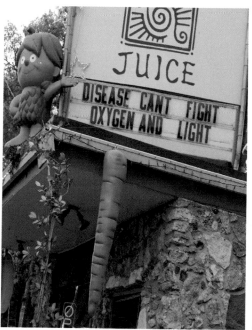

- *Eat whole foods high in nutrition,* enzymes, vitamins, and minerals with a significant quantity of chlorophyll-rich green foods, protein-rich plants, and high-water-content foods. Dark green leafy vegetables help the body detoxify and at the same time offer optimum nutrition. The fiber from the vegetables acts like an intestinal broom.

- *Drink lots of pure filtered water* every day, as well as raw vegetable juices, especially green ones. There are many filtered waters and springwaters available on the market today.

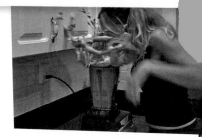

- *Eat plant foods* (like flaxseeds) containing naturally occurring omega-3 fatty acids. These are important for normal growth, help with brain repair, and support good heart health.

- *Eat a moderate yet adequate calorie intake* with low amounts of sugar exclusively from whole food sources. Sugar should be avoided by anyone dealing with cancer.

- *Eat at least 80 percent of your food raw.*

- *Exercise every day.* (More on this in just a moment.) Move that body!

- *Take enzyme, nutrient-rich superfoods* in supplement form. Superfoods are those that are nutrient-dense, like spirulina and chlorella.

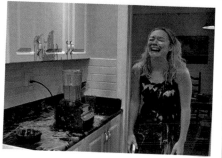

- *In addition* to all of Brenda's terrific recommendations, I take a B12 vitamin. It's the only nutrient missing from the veggie-head diet.

tip no.63

SHAKE YOUR
ass!

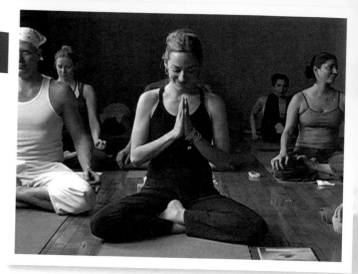

Here's an awesome statistic I learned from Dr. Brian Clement: The body heals eight times faster with exercise. Eight times! Exercise floods the body with oxygen and rids it of toxins via the lymphatic system. The body has two circulatory systems, one for blood and the other for lymph (a colorless fluid that bathes every cell in the body). The blood is lucky: It gets circulated by that pump called the heart. Lymph, on the other hand, is circulated by a pump called exercise. Many tissues depend on lymph to provide nutrients (including oxygen) and carry off wastes. If the lymph doesn't circulate, then the tissues suffocate by sitting in the stagnation of their own acidic waste products.

One of the best ways to exercise is to jump on a mini trampoline or rebounder. As you bounce, your cells get gently squeezed by the alternation of weightlessness and gravitational pull. As a result, toxins are flushed and nutrition floods your body. It's also extremely gentle on your joints. If you're too wiped out to jump, then sit and bounce or do gentle stretches.

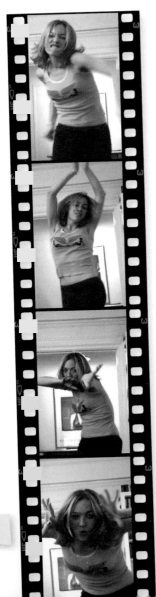

Light movement is better than no movement at all.

I can recommend lots of different types of exercise, everything from yoga to karate. But the best kind is the kind you'll actually do. So figure out what you like to do best and get moving! Let's face it, besides the physical benefits it delivers, exercise just makes you feel good. It releases endorphins and is a great overall attitude adjuster. Experts suggest we get our hearts pumping three to five times a week for about thirty-five minutes. Add some weight training to that and you're protecting yourself from bone density loss. Yup, did you know that weight-bearing exercise is the best way to fend off osteoporosis, especially once you cut back or give up the cow juice? So get out there and shake your ass, do some down dogs, buy a hula hoop, round up your posse and do some double Dutch, or hit the streets or fields for a brisk walk, gentle trot, or all-out run. You're a warrior, so start your training. If you're stuck in a hospital bed or extremely debilitated (for now), don't fret: You can still train by visualizing yourself shaking your booty! Never underestimate the mind–body connection.

TRY ALTERNATIVE
detoxing procedures

The benefits of detoxification are many. Here are just a few ways to get you flowing and glowing.

massage AND acupuncture

Both are terrific for moving blockages, stimulating energy flow, and creating better circulation and lymph drainage. Plus, they can really help you take it down a notch. If you're queasy about needles, try acupressure.

Another thought: Look for a massage therapist who uses aromatherapy as part of your session. Those powerful little herbs and petals contain oxygen molecules that get transported into the body. Different oils affect different organs; a good aromatherapist can mix a concoction tailored to your needs.

SAUNAS and steam baths

Saunas and steam baths are both excellent forms of what I call "hot box detox." Dry heat stimulates more oil-based organs like your liver and gallbladder; it also can help to melt cholesterol and plaque in your veins. Steam heat stimulates and strengthens water-based organs such as your kidneys, bladder, and lungs. Far infrared sauna therapy, which is often used at alternative healing centers as part of a regular detox program for cancer patients, penetrates the tissues of the body at a much deeper level. It's great for pulling out heavy metals and other poisons. Far infrared differs from conventional saunas in that it heats you up from the inside out and does so at much

lower temperatures, allowing you to stay in longer. I splurged for one last year and am completely in love with it. The external benefits to my skin, complexion, and even cellulite are amazing!

dry BRUSHING

Your skin is the largest organ of your body. It's said that we dump between two and five pounds of toxins per day out of our skin! Your skin needs to breathe, so dry-brush it with a natural-bristle brush (which you can find at any health food store). Dry-brushing helps keep the skin pathway clean and clear so that waste can leave the body easily. It also stimulates the lymph and helps break up my other favorite topic—cellulite. Now I bet you'll all run out and get one!

HOT baths

Not only are they incredibly calming, but hot baths are deeply therapeutic as well. Add some baking soda (make sure it's aluminum-free), sea salt, or Epsom salts—all great for pulling out heavy metals, radiation, and acids. Plus, baking soda is wonderfully alkalizing. A few additional drops of essential oils will stimulate a deeper cleanse. And don't forget the candles and music.

sleep!

Lack of sleep has devastating effects on your health. Once your final meal of the day is digested, your body diverts its energy output into cleaning and repair. This happens while you are asleep, ideally for eight hours between 10:00 p.m. and 6:00 a.m. It is therefore imperative that you finish eating three hours before going to sleep so that your body uses that precious time the right way. If sleep is cut short, the body doesn't have time to complete all the phases needed for muscle repair, memory enhancement, the release of hormones, and regulating the metabolism. Lack of sleep can also greatly affect your immune system. For the best results, try to establish regular sleeping times and avoid caffeine or alcohol. It's also important to sleep in total darkness—light leaks affect your pineal gland's production of melatonin and serotonin, the two chemicals that facilitate slumber.

{ cook well, eat well, and have fun! }

You don't have to make all the changes I'm recommending overnight. When you get your diagnosis, though, it's time to make a plan to do whatever you can to boost your immune system. It's not the time to think of living your life as if it were your last meal. ("Hey I have cancer, I deserve to eat anything I want" is not a productive attitude.) Now, this is not to say that you won't "re-tox" from time to time—we're all human beings. But if you fall off the wagon, brush yourself off and jump back on.

Be creative. Find imagination in your fridge and create art on your plate. I've included some of my standard recipes at the back of this book to help you get started. But when preparing your grub, try not to get married to someone else's exact recipes. Improvise! The best food to eat is the food you make yourself. A piece of your heart is in everything you make, so do it with joy and love. Improve your body, mind, and spirit one meal at a time.

remember:

A commonsense approach to living creates an environment where miracles can occur.

What should you eat? Food. Not too much. Mostly plants.

Consider preparing your own food as a sacred expression of creativity and self-love.

A mostly raw, vegetarian diet is loaded with enzymes—the laborers who build your body.

Creating the proper pH balance within the body is essential to vibrant health.

The best way to increase the alkalinity of your body is to adopt a vegetarian diet with a high concentration of raw foods.

By eating a diet high in chlorophyll, you dine on oxygen, the substance you need to stay alive and thrive.

Only a clean, healthy colon can absorb the nutrients from the food you eat and eliminate waste and toxins.

Unclog your colon with an enema or colonics.

When you combine food properly, the traffic in your gut moves easily.

Drink good water! Lots of it!

A diet heavy with animal products is highly acidic; acidity creates an environment for cancer cells to thrive.

Good fats are an important part of a healthy diet.

Your body heals eight times faster with exercise.

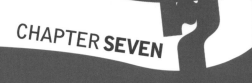

CHAPTER **SEVEN**

bald is *beautiful*

AND OTHER FACTS ABOUT FEMININITY AND FASHION

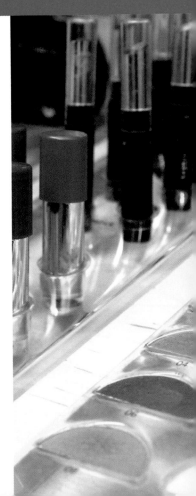

Grab your holster and six-shooter, cowgirl, it's time to confront the mirror! Walk slowly, lower your chin into your power glare, and get ready to face off. Can't you just hear the old spaghetti-western theme music playing in the background? Look yourself in the eye and say "Ta da!" (This exercise is even more rewarding when done in the nude. Gulp.) Don't worry: No matter what you see, you won't break.

It's okay to be scared, and it's okay to be vain. You're used to seeing the same girl stare back at you each day. It's a real shock when you can barely recognize yourself. You've heard this before, but I swear on John Wayne's grave, it's true: The most beautiful asset a woman can posses isn't her hair, her breasts, her soft skin, or her curvy hips, it's her imperfections. Think of the sexy, not-so-classic beauties who work their uniqueness, transforming it into success. My role models have big schnozzes, movie-screen foreheads, and gap teeth. Look beyond the mirror into the deep and soulful goddess you've become. You may be banged up and feeling like fifty cents rather than a million bucks, but remember, this body of yours is only a temporary house built to protect the righteous Aphrodite within. Worship her.

{ follicle freak-out }

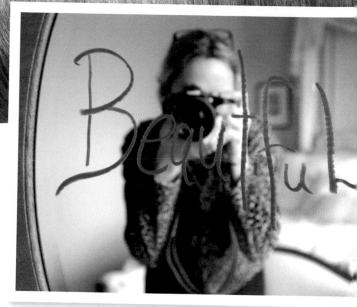

The first thing I asked when I found out I had cancer was, "Will I lose my hair?" The second question was "Will I die?"—second! That's how important my hair was to me. I'm not alone. For a lot of women, their locks are their defining feature, a symbol of femininity, sexual power, even fertility! For some, losing their hair can be even more traumatic than losing their breasts. Why? Because the change is obvious, and even if you don't feel sick, without hair, you look it.

My fine and stringy hair had always given me stress. I didn't have bad hair days, I had bad hair years. I cringe when I look at the collection of awkward cuts and colors displayed on our family photo mantel (at my mother's insistence). Why is it that every time I got restless in my life, I got bangs?

My job only exacerbated the situation. Always having to change hair color for roles took a toll on my tender shoots. I remember one jet-black dye job for an episode of *Law & Order*. My grandmother had just returned from her weekly fluff-and-clip trip to the "beauty parlor." Innocently, I thought it would be nice to give the ol' gal a compliment. "Wow, Grandma, you look so beautiful. Stunning!"

"I weesh I cood zay the zame for you," she squawked back in her thick Colombian accent. The woman was never one to mince words.

My sister, on the other hand—now, that girl has hair! Thick, curly come-hither locks. I tried everything to replicate her mane. Perms, treatments, you name it. I even tried clip-on extensions. I figured, celebrities got away with it, so why couldn't I? Big mistake! Case in point: One particularly hot makeout session turned frigid when my date tried to run his fingers through my faux strands. One minute my golden locks cascaded down my back; the next they lay sprawled in his hand like a dead ferret with a clip glued to its head. The guy had no idea what hit him. We laughed about it, but that was the end of that. Apparently I was too high-maintenance. What? Me? I own, like, two beauty products and a stick of deodorant! My first attempt at being "girlie" and I fell flat on my face. Like all handicaps, bad hair forced me to play up my other strengths. My sense of humor kept the bees buzzing toward the honey.

Despite all that, I did not want to lose my locks to cancer.

{ confidence loss }

As it turned out, I didn't lose my hair, but I did lose my confidence. Even though I had no visible signs of cancer on the outside, on the inside I felt flawed and different. I still recognized the girl in the mirror, but I sensed that a part of her was gone. Cancer had dulled my sparkle; in my mind, my body had betrayed me. How could I be confident when I felt like a walking skull and crossbones?

HAVE A SHAVING PARTY!

Heidi:
When it starts to go, get it gone fast! Shaving or cutting your hair as soon as it starts to fall out will help you maintain some modicum of control over a difficult transition. Use this as an opportunity to try out those kicky short styles you were too scared to try before!

PROFILE:
SHARON BLYNN

sharon's icon:

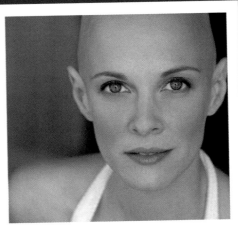

AGE: 35

HAIR COLOR: None (stubble available with three to four days' notice!)

EYES: Hazel

HEIGHT: 5'10"

WEIGHT: 120

HOMETOWN: New York City

OCCUPATION: Actor, writer, activist, founder of Bald Is Beautiful

FAVORITE SAYING: "Always smile from the inside out!" (My life motto.)

BEST TIP: "If you're feeling helpless, help someone." —Burmese human rights advocate Aung San Suu Kyi

{ au naturel }

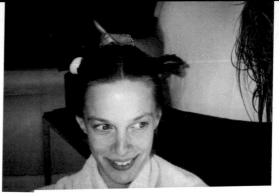

Inspired by her experience with ovarian cancer and chemotherapy-induced hair loss, Sharon created BaldIsBeautiful.org, a Web site that seeks to help women embrace their baldness with a sense of adventure and pride. Though Sharon is in remission, she continues to shave her gleaming, smooth crown as a badge of courage. As she sees it, her lack of hair reminds her that she's a survivor, and her scars have become beauty marks. "You simply have to adjust your thinking," she points out.

Sharon:

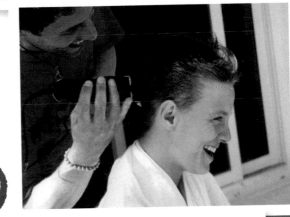

I had long hair for nearly my entire life. I was a hippie chick, my flowing locks symbols of flower power, peace, and love. I couldn't imagine cutting my hair, ever. But suddenly diagnosed with ovarian cancer in the summer of 2000, I faced losing my hair—all of it. How could I say good-bye to something I considered so central to my identity? I decided to make the process fun, turning my fear into a positive, empowering choice to reinvent myself. I conquered it in phases.

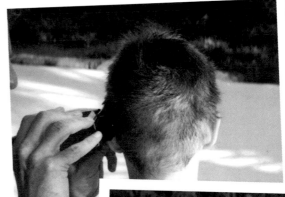

Phase One: short haircut, donate locks to Wigs for Kids. When the day came for my haircut, I was in too much pain to go anywhere. My twin Elisa (monozygotes rule!) drove to the salon, and apparently it went something like this: "Sharon started chemotherapy and needs her hair cut now." Cut to haircut houseccall. Smiling with nervous anticipation, I tied

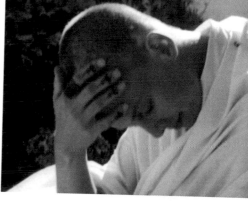

my hair into pigtails. Two quick snips from Michelle, my hairstylist, and my long hair was no more. The two of us burst into teary-eyed smiles, and hugged tightly. My dread was overshadowed, banished, by this loving gift of Michelle's time, making what could've been a somber occasion into one of my life's most special events. This was the beginning of my coming into myself in a way I'd never anticipated. There was much more to come (out, that is) nine days later.

All good hairs must eventually come to a split end, and so the surreal part of the process began.

I'd wake up with mounds of hair on my pillow. When I ran my fingers through my hair, large clumps appeared in my palms. I stared at them, covered in my own hair, feeling helpless. It was everywhere—on my bed, the floor, in the sink, the kitchen. Everywhere I went, I left a trail of expelled hair. The worst part was washing it. Bad idea. Hair all over me, all over the bathtub, and now it was wet and sticky and didn't just easily wipe away. I felt I was being tarred and feathered! Finally, a mere head nod that extricated a mutinous cascade of hair brought on Phase Two of my transformation: the electric razor. I sat down, took a deeeeeeep breath: Wirrrrrrrrr!

No turning back, I was a bald chick. It was then that I began to see myself in a whole new way. As I embraced my own chemo-induced baldness with a sense of adventure, I was shocked by the overwhelmingly positive response I received, especially because I had been so consumed with anxiety and fear about losing my hair in the first place. The experience sparked in me a fierce desire to dispel the stigma that is associated with hair loss due to chemotherapy— or any other hair loss conditions, for that matter. I wanted to do something to expand social concepts of what constitutes beauty and femininity, and to promote the idea that

women are not the sum of their body parts. With or without hair, breasts, or reproductive organs, we are spiritually whole and perfect.

FAUX PAS!

When an out-of-control heckler shouts, "Nice haircut!" politely respond, "Thanks, my oncologist styled it!" Open mouth, insert foot.

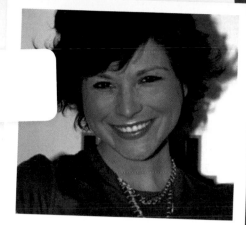

PROFILE:
DIEM BROWN

AGE: 25¼, and determined to make it to a dollar one day!

HAIR COLOR: Depends on my mood. It's been blond, pink, red, red with black streaks, and honey. Now it's dark brown.

EYES: Brown with green flecks. I'll not give up the flecks!

HEIGHT: 5'5½"—once again it's all in the details!

WEIGHT: More than a buck, less than two. That's as detailed as I'm getting with this question.

HOMETOWN: Army brat, but the roots I did manage to put down were in Roswell, Georgia. I consider myself a Southern Gal!

OCCUPATION: Founder and executive director of Live for the Challenge (www.l4tc.com), the first and only medical gift registry—aka "my heart and soul!"

FAVORITE SAYING: "Grin and bear it!"

BEST TIP: Do everything! People always look back and say, "I wish I had done that or this." You never hear someone say, "I wish I hadn't done everything I wanted to do."

tip no.66

WIG IT out!

My pal Diem is also an ovarian cancer survivor. She is known for her role on *MTV's Real World/Road Rules Challenge: Fresh Meat*. And let me tell you, this girl is a spitfire! One month after losing one of her ovaries, several lymph nodes, and part of a fallopian tube, she headed to Australia for five weeks of intense physical training and endurance tests. She survived everything from hanging on to a fake alligator while it thrashed her around like a rinse cycle gone mad to dangling fifty feet in the air while blindfolded. She even had to swim with sharks! Diem did all this with cancer. "It was the best experience of my life," she says.

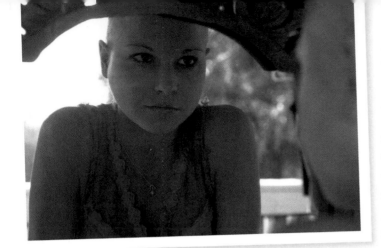

"I was able to prove to myself that cancer wouldn't hold me back."

Still, while swimming with sharks was par for the course for Diem, losing her hair was a real struggle.

Diem:

For me, my changing image in the mirror was a reality check I was not ready to handle. I had a tendency to run from things that scared me, and death had always been at the top of my "Oh fudge!" list. Every time hair would fall out I kept thinking, *Why can't I stop this?* Looking in the mirror was a constant reminder that my cancer was real and I was sick. My image scared me. Running wasn't going to make it go away. It took me awhile to realize that while I had no control over what was happening to my physical appearance, I did have control over things in my life, like making myself feel better.

My first wig-shopping experience was not as fun as I thought it would be. I hated being in a wig store and seeing the tape and Styrofoam heads, so I left and went for frozen yogurt instead. But once I got used to the "wig life," my girlfriends convinced me to try out some "fun wigs." We made a day of it. We went to this hole-in-the-wall wig shop and asked to see all wigs under $30. These models came with names like Candy, Fire, and Ginger. We had a blast with the crazy names and looks. Appropriately, the pink short one was named Bubbles. Whenever I would don that one, I only answered to Bubbles.

My girlfriends weren't about to let me have all the fun. They wanted in on the party, too. So we threw "wig nights." We would all dress up in my wigs and go out on the town. The guys loved it! At the same time, seeing my healthy friends with wigs on helped me get over the stigma I had about wearing a wig. So I say "wig it out" and let your friends join in the fun! It'll help you get used to your new Styrofoam head life.

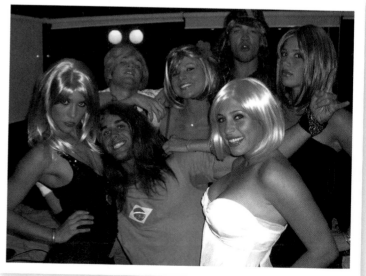

HELP YOURSELF TO A
blond flip or a pink beauty

Speaking of Styro heads, my friend Jackie had a Rockette kick line of wigs positioned on top of her 1950s-style living room bar. She was quite the cancer hostess! You could either help yourself to a nip from the crystal bourbon decanter or pet the blond flip. Jackie had a wig for every day and every mood. One day she was a hot blonde; the next, Mary Tyler Moore. Like Diem, she also cruised around in a pink beauty. Of all her strands, this one was the coolest! Pink really does wonders for your complexion and your spirits. I was inspired to make my own pink wig purchase, and let me tell you, Brian loves it (but that's another story!).

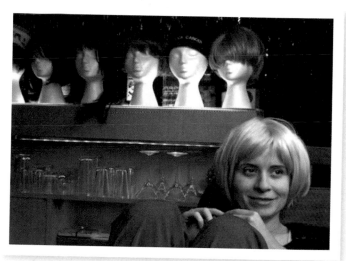

Jackie:

My first real wig-shopping experience was a nightmare. My insurance company told me I would be reimbursed $800 for wigs, so I went to an upscale wig shop and went to town. I found out later that I would be reimbursed in the amount of zero dollars. The good news was that I had a top-of-the-line wig collection.

Damaged goods is a term I often used to describe how I felt about myself. I grew up in Synanon, the California commune (cult) where addict parents cleaned up and kids were required to have bald heads. It was mortifying. When I left Synanon, I burned the photos to forget. So on top of facing all the struggles that come with cancer, the last thing I needed was to lose was my hair—again! It was one of the few things about my looks that I liked and was confident about. Growing it back was at least a year of a terrible Afro. I mean Afro! No one told me that it would grow back differently.

I know some women choose to rock the bald head. Maybe it's a way for them to express that they are not letting cancer consume their lives. I wear wigs. Aside from the reasons above, it's my way of making it fun. Wigs made me feel attractive again.

One of my favorites was long, blond, and luscious. With one stroke of the brush, I looked like one of those women who spend an hour blowing and styling their hair every day. It was super-blond—

one of the only colors I never dyed my hair. The style was on the sexy side.

Still, my all-time favorite was my Pink Beauty. It was my first playful wig. Wearing it, I felt a little more like my old self. I went out a little more. Most comments from strangers were positive. Of course I got some strange looks, too, but in hindsight maybe that's part of what made me feel more like me.

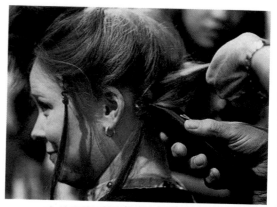

Like Jackie, my friend Melissa managed to make the wigalicious life work for her. Both these posse members reveal that while it can be traumatic to lose your hair, you can still look your best, thanks to all the options out there.

Melissa:

Through CancerCare I received a "hair prosthesis" donated by Rodolfo Valentin, a salon owner in New York. Because I had long (red) hair, Rodolfo suggested that we use my own hair. This was actually a great thing, because I didn't have to wait around for my hair to fall out. I was in control, not the cancer. Rodolfo shaved my hair, made a mold of my head, and two weeks later I had my hair back. It fit on my head like a glove. To have this done usually costs about $5,000, so it was very generous of him to make the donation. I wore the wig almost daily through my first treatment and then again when I relapsed. I had fancy scarves and hats that I would wear on the really hot summer days, but for the most part I never left home without it. I even made it through my ten-year reunion without anyone noticing that I was wearing a wig. Having this prosthesis

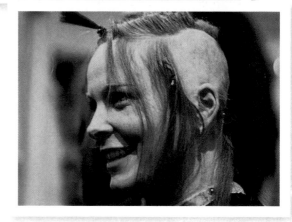

made a huge difference throughout the ordeal by helping me maintain my vanity. Just because you are a cancer patient doesn't mean you have to look like one!

"Resolve to take fate by the throat and shake a living out of her."
—LOUISA MAY ALCOTT, AUTHOR

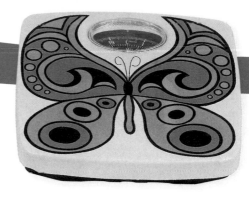

tip no.68

THROW OUT
the scale

It's the enemy! Whether you think you're too small or too big, the saying "There is power in numbers" is all too true when it comes to the scale monster. Why do we constantly try to shrink ourselves to feel bigger and better? Or layer on bulky clothes to look "normal"? I remember the stinging words of the cool girl in sixth grade: "Kristin's so skinny she has to run around in the shower to get wet." She was the "It girl" in the prepubescent pack. I can still see her feathered Farrah Fawcett hair flying up and down as she hunted me in her Gloria Vanderbilt jeans. I sported Wrangler's.

We all want to fit in. Even in my thirties I'm tempted by the pressures of the cool crowd at times. But while you're undergoing cancer treatments with all their debilitating side effects, you don't have to keep up appearances.

Though chemo never peeled off my pounds, my self-prescribed radical detoxes did. During my first fast I went from a size 8 (normal) to a size 0 (emaciated). That's when an interesting and very dangerous thing happened. I became thrilled! A fake and temporary confidence emerged, and it was the worst thing that could've happened. In my mind I looked great. Go cancer! Of course, hiding underneath my newly purchased style (I overindulged in some serious shopping therapy) were a set of deflated pancake boobs and a rickety skeleton. But no matter. Finally, I was really skinny!

As with most diets, the results were temporary. I packed the weight back on and then some. I felt so blue. The roller-coaster ride I went on with my weight actually bothered me more than the cancer. At the end of the day, I was ashamed of myself for playing the super-skinny game. For many of us, a healthy weight is not the one we're constantly chasing. It's the one we're at when we say, "Oh, if I could just lose five or ten pounds . . ."

Erin:

After I found out I had cancer, my mom and I left the hospital and had lunch. While I was walking through the neighborhood where we ate, I noticed a spa and I thought, *Maybe I'll get an eyebrow wax.* Then I immediately thought, I should be crying or praying and instead I'm contemplating an eyebrow wax.

Society sets this impossible standard for how cancer patients are supposed to act and think. We're expected to become very centered and sane. I found that whole idea to be a big burden. It's way too much pressure! Every time I think, I look fat in these jeans—a completely natural thought—am I supposed to also feel bad for the fact that I have cancer and I still don't have perspective? At the end of the day, we're still women and we have the same thoughts as other women. When I'm prescribed a new medication, I think: *Is this going to make me gain weight?*

Some might think these thoughts are un-PC, but I think they're a perfectly natural and normal reaction for a woman. Even with a cancer diagnosis, it's okay to still want to look good. Sure, you have to let go of some things, but there's no cancer "do and don't" list.

Jackie:

I struggled with my weight my entire life, and when I went into remission the first time, I worked really hard to get the extra steroid weight off and keep it off. Then I relapsed, hit the 'roids even harder, and gained another twenty pounds within a few weeks. Not to seem vain, but when I feel ugly, bald, fat, and like shit, it's hard to focus on getting back into the swing of life. As my strength builds, so will my weight loss efforts. The better I feel about myself, the quicker I'll be able to put all this cancer crap behind me.

{ titties, knockers, ta tas, boozangas, boobies }

"Dear God, bless Mom, Dad, Leslie, Grandma, and Uncle Chase and Aunt Judy, and please send me some boobs. Amen." Like most young girls, I was focused on growing up, fast! When I turned nine, I was ready to turn ten, and so on. I had been watching and waiting as all the other girls were developing left and right, leaving me in the dust. Coming from a family of big-breasted women, I was both nervous and excited to get my own set—although maybe not quite so big. So when my grandmother told me that if I ate my spinach I'd get big boozangas like her, I made sure to gooble up at least half of what she shoveled onto my plate, just to be safe. Every day I'd wake up and peek, but all I'd see were two peas under wallpaper. It was pathetic.

My prize possession was my training bra. My mom had purchased it at Bloomingdale's and placed it strategically behind the bunny in my Easter basket so as not to embarrass me. (If my little sister had spotted it, she no doubt would have asked *What's that for?*) I immediately put it on for a test drive, only to be humiliated by a pack of bullies in the girls' locker room at school.

Finally my breasts kicked in, and so did my period. I was in heaven, a real woman. My parents even took me out for some rite-of-passage celebratory pizza, a "P" party they called it—awkward but special. The next year the braces came off, and Peter Andrews, the captain of the lacrosse team, copped a feel in Spanish class. That was it, the defining moment. That little squeeze changed everything. For the first time in my life I was desired.

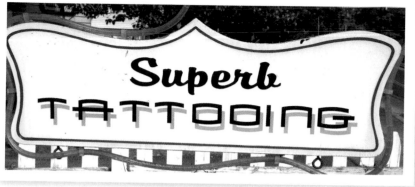

Would losing my breasts take that away? What would I do: implant, no implant? One boob and proud? What about the nipple—does that go, too? And if so, then what? A cool tattoo of a flower or a dragon? So many questions, so many options! Another reason I am lucky to have my posse is that in sharing our many different stories and perspectives, it's clear the issues we discuss are universal.

Allison:

Losing my breasts was an entirely different experience from losing my hair. It was really, really, really hard, and to be honest it still is. On the days leading to my surgery, I completely lost it. I was so scared that I was making the wrong decision. I had to do a lot of research and deep soul searching to come to terms with my decision. But once the surgery was over, it was a relief. There's no turning back now, I thought. Even though it's hard sometimes to face the dramatic changes my body has endured, I'm proud of my decision. I am thankful to have my life.

Women who lose their breast or breasts to cancer have a few options. First, they can opt to have reconstruction or not. Second, they can choose to have implants put in, or they can choose to do an autologous tissue reconstruction, which entails using the tissue from another part of your own body to create a breast.

The tissue reconstruction was not an option for me because I am very thin, especially after the weight I lost on chemo. However, I wanted reconstruction, so I chose to have implants. At the time of my mastectomy, my surgeon put what are called expanders underneath the muscles in my chest to expand the tissue and prepare it for the implant. I worked with my surgeon to pick the implants that we thought would be best for my body. I wanted to come as close as possible to the look that my breasts had pre-surgery. After about four months my surgeon switched the expanders out for the permanent implants. The mastectomy wasn't too painful—uncomfortable, but not entirely debilitating. And the implant exchanges didn't hurt at all. The initial surgery makes your chest completely numb, which on a day-to-day basis is a bummer, but when it comes to having surgery it's great!

I am still in the process of deciding what to do about nipple reconstruction. At first I thought I would just go without. It actually sounded kind of nice to not have to worry about nipples showing through my clothes ever again. But lately I've been having second thoughts. I'd prefer not to be reminded of my mastectomy every time I look in the mirror. I am hoping that the appearance of nipples will lessen the reminder and allow me to feel a little more normal on a day-to-day basis. As with the breast reconstruction, I have a few choices as to how I could reconstruct my nipples. The surgeons can use the tissue on my breast to pucker the skin and create a nipple, or they can transplant a small amount of tissue from somewhere else on my body. The areola will then have to be tattooed on to create the color variance.

Cancer took away so many things that I identified with my beauty as a woman: hair, breasts, eyebrows, eyelashes, and even my fingernails and toenails. It's an interesting transition. I thought it would all be devastating, but it wasn't.

I began to focus on the beauty of living far more than I focused on my external beauty. The strength and love cancer brought into my life actually made me feel more beautiful than ever.

Now my hair and nails are growing back, but my hair is different. My once stick-straight blond hair is coming in curly and a tad darker than it was. When I look in the mirror, I see a different person than I saw a year ago. It's not only the physical changes that are different; it's also the person I have become. When I look at pictures of myself taken before my diagnosis, I hardly recognize the girl I see. I will always miss my body the way it was before cancer, but I will forever be proud of the body that I have now because it symbolizes my battle and my courage.

tip no.**69**

SPLURGE ON A PRETTY, LACY BRA THAT BRINGS OUT YOUR
inner sex goddess

New boobs or no boobs, you still deserve to feel lacy and special. Cleavage confidence on the inside is what really makes you stand out from all the other showgirls at the soiree. And ladies: Get a bra fitting!

Allison:
Bra shopping post-mastectomy was not a fun experience, to say the least! My breasts were different, and I felt differ-ent about them. I was lucky in that my doctor was able to get them very close to my original size. However, the difference became very obvious to me when I tried to wear my old bras. One day I put on one of my pre-mastectomy bras. I wore it all day, no problem, or so I thought. When I came home that evening, I real-ized that the underwire of the bra had been digging into my breasts throughout

the day. I was near bleeding, but had no idea because the mastectomy had left me without any feeling. Needless to say, I now have to be very careful when I select bras to fit "the new me."

Thankfully, there are experts out there to help you find the perfect bra for the new you. One is Lisa Cole, a lingerie-fitting and mastectomy-form expert who helps women shop for a bra after either a lumpectomy or a mastectomy. She has a great way of thinking about the first bra-shopping experience post-surgery: "It's about celebrating the fact that you are a survivor. And I often say: Girlfriend, you should even buy a thong! If you were a crazy, sexy, hot mama before, there's no need to change." Here are a few tips from Lisa on how to find the perfect crazy sexy bra:

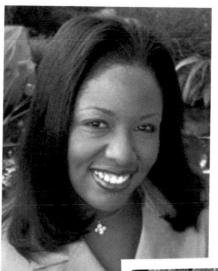

Bra guru Lisa Cole

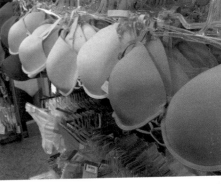

- **Get advice from an expert.** Eight out of ten women are wearing the wrong size bra. If you've had a mastectomy or lumpectomy, your challenge is even greater. Make an appointment with a certified specialist for a fitting. Many department stores and some pharmacies provide this service, free of charge. And consider bringing a friend who can encourage you and help make this a positive experience.

- **Put a pocket in it.** Don't limit yourself to mastectomy bras with sewn-in pockets. A seamstress can sew a pocket into any bra. Just make sure the prosthesis fits properly in the bra in order to give you the proper shape and comfort.

- **When selecting a bra, think Crazy sexy hot mama!** Buy at least one sexy, lacy number. This can help you feel feminine and beautiful from within. Lingerie supports us, shapes us, and allows us to be comfortable in our skin. Clip pictures of trendy styles from magazines and bring them to your appointment.

- **Buy the right kind of bra.** In addition to making sure you're wearing the right size bra, make sure you buy the right style. With the right style and fit, no one will know you've had a mastectomy or lumpectomy. Fill your lingerie drawer with bras for every outfit, including bras that are strapless, convertible, contour (for T-shirts and knits), seamless, non-underwires, push-ups (great for plunging necklines), and sports bras.

- **Make sure you know what your insurance covers.** Before you go bra shopping, check with your health insurer.

LIPSTICK CAN MOVE MOUNTAINS
so get a cancer makeover

We've all heard of the importance of inner beauty. Once again, easier said than done. Yes, I want to be pretty on the inside . . . but I also want to look good. Is that too much to ask? Don't get me wrong, inner beauty is a powerful weapon in any arsenal. But sometimes concealer and a tube of gloss can really help you be the kind and confident person you strive to be. We're all so offended by construction worker catcalls, but it's even more offensive when they stop. You just may need a little buffing to make you feel like you're still in the game. Here's some advice that will keep the dogs howling and resurrect your shine:

Go get your hair styled, your face sparkled, and throw in a mani and a pedi for good measure. Just because we're sick doesn't mean we have to look it.

I know this is a stitch-and-bitch cancer hens book, but I have included one honorary male member. My friend Ramy Gafni proves that a little lipstick can move mountains! Ramy is an amazing makeup artist, author, and cancer survivor. I met him at a cancer fund-raiser at Joe's Salon in New Milford, Connecticut (the hot spot for haircuts in my hometown). Ramy had just released his book *Beauty Therapy: The Ultimate Guide to Looking and Feeling Great While Living with Cancer*. At the salon that day, he was giving free makeovers to cancer patients. Women of all ages in various stages of their treatment crowded the shop, eager for some beauty tips.

RAMY'S *story*

I was a happy-go-lucky makeup artist with a career on the fast track. I loved my job and my life. Then I was diagnosed with non-Hodgkin's lymphoma and suddenly the good-looking chic New Yorker I was used to seeing in the mirror disappeared and was replaced by a bald, puffy

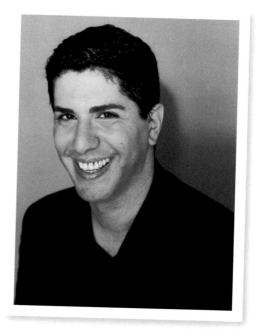

guy with really dark undereye circles and a pasty complexion. At the time, I was working as makeup director at a top Fifth Avenue salon where the pressure to look good was intense. Thankfully, as a makeup artist I knew what to do to counteract the physical side effects of chemo and radiation treatments. A little concealer around my eyes covered up the dark circles and made me look more rested than

chapter seven in review:

remember:

Cancer scars are beauty marks.

Women are not the sum of their body parts.

Live the wig life! Have fun with wigs, even pink ones!

Throw out the scale. Take a break from the weight game.

Get a bra fitting.

Cancer Babes with breast cancer: Explore your reconstruction options.

Lipstick can move mountains.

Indulge in regular beauty rituals.

bandage or bondage:
DATING, SEX, MARRIAGE, BABIES

It's not surprising that sex isn't always at the top of a Cancer Babe's to-do list after her diagnosis and treatment! In some cases we're hurt, freaked out, and feeling like aliens in a foreign body. And let's be real: Dating is treacherous with or without cancer. Depending on your treatment saga, getting involved and bringing someone into your cancer world can be intimidating for you both. Body image baggage, missing parts, infertility, a lack of confidence, and all the other stuff I've talked about in the last chapters can put a damper on your inner Venus.

Survivors often find that there is a big difference between dating post- and pre-cancer. No matter what, cancer changes you. When you're recovering from trauma, intimacy can make you feel raw and vulnerable. Cancer treatments can cause embarrassing symptoms like vaginal dryness and the emotional turbulence of premature menopause. You may not be able to swing from the trapeze like you used to. Certain activities or positions that made you light up in the past may now shut down the whole the system.

But there are lots of ways to get the engine started. Be creative: You have a new body now, so why not try something new to please it?

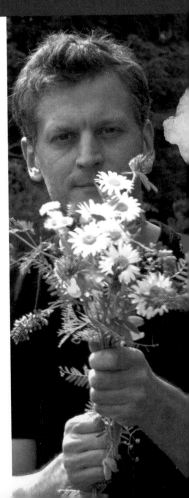

Change the lens, flip the script; it's normal to feel like a mangled mess. Validate your thoughts by letting them out, but don't let them rule the roost! If you don't come to terms with how you've changed and who you are now, it will be harder to let someone else accept, love, and even touch you. This is true if you're married, dating, or even just looking at the menu with no intention of ordering.

As clichéd as it sounds, love and affection with the right person can nurture a healing that reaches beyond your cancer baggage and into the foundation of your well-being. We all have old wounds. Once we deal with the upheaval that cancer churns up, those old bruises can finally begin to heal.

Choose to go forward with abandon. Cancer can ignite an inner revolution and sexual liberation—if we let it. "I'm a supernova-ass-kicking survivor, sexier than ever and ready to tango in the sheets." Hell yeah! You are stronger and wiser and all grown up now. Stoke the fires and let your inner stripper rip. Even if all you feel up to is lighting some candles and cuddling, turn it on. Don't sever a portion of your womanhood.

Cancer helps us to go deeper, appreciate relationships more, and even create healthier role models for ourselves and our children.

Open your mind to the possibilities of your life. Remember, you're a cancer survivor, physically, mentally, and spiritually!

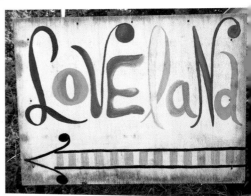

{ from hunted to quarantined }

Après the awkward years, I morphed into "the cool girlfriend." High school parents loved me. I was a good girl with manners and proper upbringing. What a smoke-and-mirrors game I had going! The parents of my high school sweetheart(s) had no idea how much hellfire and trouble was in me. I ached for love. My head was focused on boys 24/7. I knew how to wrangle them. I was voted class flirt and most likely to get divorced! I didn't know it then, but thanks to my many emotional bruises and scars I was setting the stage for a major co-dependency problem. I wound up being a professional girlfriend.

Until I was diagnosed I was barely single. I didn't know how to let a casual dinner date be just that. Dinner to me usually took about six months to digest! By the time I realized I wanted out, it was usually too late. It took a big lie or escapade to extract myself from the relationship. "My missing twin has just been found in Guam. I need to relocate in order to build this long-lost relationship." I would gnaw off my own arm just to sneak out and be alone.

Then I was alone. Very single, very alone, and very sick. Cancer changed everything. Not that I wanted a knight on a white horse to sweep me up and make it all go away. My sex drive had slammed into reverse, and my little black book was in the deep freeze. Frankly, my only thought was not *Will I have the white picket fence dream?* but rather *Will I make it through this?*

Looking back, being alone was the best thing for me. I dropped the bullshit and got real with myself immediately. Instead of getting to know someone else, I got to know me. I found out who I was without the mirror of a man telling me who he thought I was. It was awesome! I even stopped shaving my legs for a few months. Wow, was I coming into my own.

When I was ready to hit the market again, I decided to be risqué and freelance. I wanted to test the waters, sample the appetizers, and nibble some dessert. I had no idea what it would be like, and I was both scared and strangely centered. The best thing I ever did was to do it sober. No booze whatsoever. Beer goggles were such a part of the pre-cancer years that I figured it was time for some clear judgment. How many times had I tried my darndest to lure someone into liking me without even considering whether or not he was actually worth the effort? I needed to like him, not just having company. The only problem was that since I wasn't going to bars or hanging out with the party crowd anymore, I had little access to guys. Or did I?

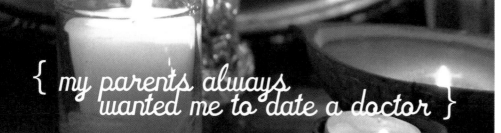

{ my parents always wanted me to date a doctor }

My first date after the scarlet letter C branding was with one of my liver specialists! Total Madonna moment (because he actually helped me get through a lot of medical red tape). I had never seen a specialist before. He had a strange name. It sounded Transylvanian. I pictured him as old and hairy with pudgy little fingers that would make me squirm when they examined my wounded liver. Maybe he was obsessed with livers? Perhaps he even ate them, delighting in their taste and texture as each well-understood morsel slid down his gruesome throat. I couldn't get these twisted fantasies out of my mind as I nervously waited for his nurse to call my name. Much to my surprise, he wasn't Hannibal Lecter. He was actually quite snappy and handsome. Oh, great—and here I'd worn my granny panties, no makeup, and a hairstyle straight out of a White Snake video. But I guess I was still able to muster up some charm.

The next hour was frightening, funny, and truly human. He peppered me with personal questions that went well beyond what my liver was up to. I wasn't sure if he was feeling me out until he started feeling me up! Since when do you get a breast exam by your liver specialist? He started over the bra but it was so padded we both laughed. Of course I was mortified because I hadn't shaved my armpits. "Um, I haven't shaved in a while—I'm staying with my parents, and the razor in the guest bathroom is rusty." Why was I telling him this? His response? "Note to self: Hair growth normal." He was cute and funny.

During the ultrasound I asked him what he saw, figuring he'd be like every other doctor and tell me, *Nothing*. "Do you want to see?" he asked. Yes! He sat next to me and turned the little screen my way. Little white speckles moved across the surface of my liver as he rubbed the camera along my belly. There they were. I finally had a picture—and apparently a date!

After I fired him (so that I could date him), we spent many sunsets zooming around in his sports car, and I felt like a weight was lifted. The best part about the relationship was that

I didn't have to deal with the awkward "outing myself" experience. Because even when dudes say it doesn't matter, it does. It matters to them and to everyone in their inner circle. "Wow, that's tough. Are you sure you want to get involved with that?" Trust me; I've heard it, and so will you. Every crazy thing that crosses your mind crosses theirs. Some are man enough to face the unknown. Others are still boys—and that's okay, too, by the way. The liver specialist made me feel alive and attractive. We played around for a few months and then I got a whiff of the four-letter L-word, freaked out, and took off. There was only room for one serious thing in my life, and at that point cancer filled the slot.

{ my second date and first official "outing" }

Michael was a drop-dead-gorgeous acupuncturist. Okay, so I was still getting involved with healer types (can you say Daddy, God, savior complex?), but at least this time I wasn't one of his patients. Blind dates generally suck; this one was a total score! Michael was kind, spiritual, and downright delicious. Maybe I should have told him upfront, but I just didn't have the guts. Actually, I was petrified. So I decided to take it really slow. If he was worth it, I'd drop the bomb when the time was right. In my mind it would be easier to tell him after we got to know each other better. But then again if he stopped calling, I'd be crushed.

Michael must have known that I had something to confess. "What are you thinking?"

he'd innocently ask as my gaze drifted into a glassy-eyed netherworld. Oh, just admiring the way the sun is caressing your tender face as I FANTASIZE ABOUT DYING AND LEAVING YOU WITH A HOUSE FULL OF MOTHERLESS CHILDREN. "Nothing and everything," I'd say. The time to get honest was lurking around the corner. It was torturous! The thought of the "I have cancer" chitchat gave me the feeling you get at the top of the roller coaster, the moment before the big free fall begins. I hate that moment! I'd rather jab a syringe full of Windex in my heart than say those three words. Sometimes being sick really sucks.

Weeks turned into months of courting, dinners, movies, and everything else that goes with falling for someone. We weren't exclusive, but it seemed like it was heading in that direction—at least from my perspective. Finally one day I just couldn't take it anymore. I was tired of my "dirty" little secret; it was time to come clean. "There's something I've wanted to tell you, but I'm really scared. It's not a big deal, but at first it will seem like one until I explain it. I have cancer." I waited for the blood to drain from his face as he made a mad dash to the nearest EXIT sign, but he didn't budge. He stayed and listened. It was over, I had told him, and now the ball was in his court. Regardless of his response I was relieved. "So what. We'll deal with it, it's okay," he said. What? Oh my God, he's perfect!

But then the other shoe dropped. "I have something to tell you, too. I'm kinda gay." Okay, I definitely didn't see that one coming! "Kinda gay" meant kinda both, kinda unsure, and kinda thinking about going back to his ex, Paul, but I could come, too, if I wanted. Though I strive to be open-minded, down deep I'm a pretty old-fashioned one-guy-at-a-time girl. Paul was not a part of my equation. Still, the experience of hanging out with a really cool guy who accepted my situation was ultimately healing for me. Even though he pitched for both teams, he made me feel like a vixen and a winner. Gold trophy!

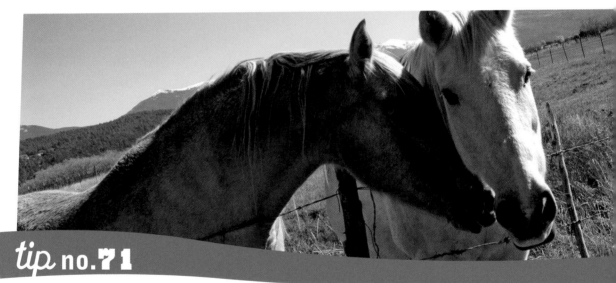

tip no.71

BE STRAIGHTFORWARD WITH *your partner*

You'll know when the time is right. Tell him your situation and don't fret. Some days you feel good; other days you get hit and dragged by the cancer train. If he can accept this and stand by your side—or better yet, jump in the trenches with you—then he's a keeper.

How many dates should you go on before telling someone that you're a survivor? There is no right or wrong answer to this question. Trust the voice inside you to let you know when the time is right. That little voice is awfully wise and too often ignored!

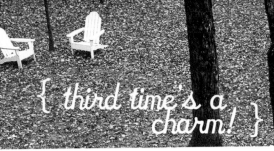

{ third time's a charm! }

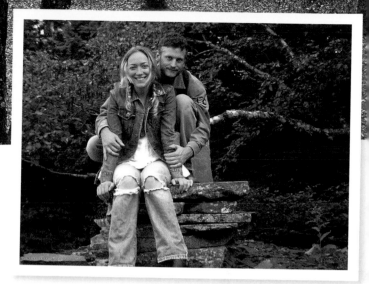

Then there was Brian . . . "Hi, gorgeous." "Hi." How long had it been since someone called me gorgeous? Cancer certainly didn't make me feel like a prize. Brian and I met through friends years ago. I remember thinking he was cute, but at the time I was taken and he was a drummer, a recipe for disaster. For ten years we'd run into each other on and off. A quick hello and a "Hey, how ya been?" But that's where it started and ended. It wasn't until I got diagnosed that I learned what Brian really did for a living. He was a writer and a film editor. Hmm, creative gents have always been a major turn-on, especially when they're jackasses! Luckily, Brian wasn't a jackass, plus I had done some maturing by then so the jerk factor had lost its appeal.

About six months into my film (and my diagnosis), I asked Brian to help me shoot and edit my project. Pretty soon we were working together all the time, documenting my journey with cancer. Sixteen-hour editing sessions were filled with creativity, playfulness, and lots of goofing around. Though I fought it at first, I was falling for the guy. It wasn't until one particular doctor's appointment that I realized how deep my feelings had become. Tough medical stuff became even harder to hear because I wanted to protect him from the information. But how could I shelter my cameraman and still tell my story? Remember, he was filming it all for The Learning Channel.

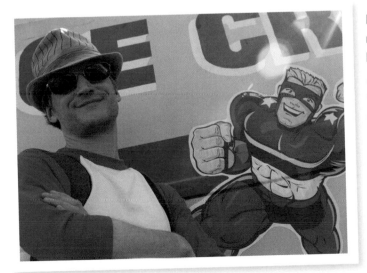

So I tried to break up with him. Brilliant! The first balanced, normal, talented, laid-back, and loving guy to come around in, like, *forever*—and I called it off! "It's over; you have your whole life ahead of you, find a healthy chick and be normal. This is my burden and I like you too much to bring you into the fold."

He refused. "Nope. I love you and I'm staying. Let's take it one day at a time and work with what we've got, okay?" Okay!

Am I even ready to date? Maybe it would be a good distraction for me. But love, actually falling in love. I don't know if my heart could handle the infectious nature of love. I am already consumed in my struggle for recovery. I guess I am just petrified of getting hurt. But he knows. Wow, he knows and he is still interested. Not that a man is going to make it all go away or make me feel complete.

But this man sure makes the dark days a little brighter.

Here was a man who knew it all, every detail, and he wasn't running. It was *freaky*. So we kept working together, and I no longer slept on the couch.

Later I realized that our creative union was healing for me. Brian provided space for me to process my disease in the edit room. Over the years it has been him, above anyone else in my life, who has helped me to blossom in the face of cancer and to make peace with the unknown. Not that we haven't had our bumps along the way. But I can actually say that the best thing to happen to me as a result of cancer was getting to know and eventually marry my soul mate.

{ getting hitched }

My wedding was the best day of my life. "Ya wanna make God laugh? Tell Her your plans." Great saying, right? Well I could definitely hear Her chuckling as I walked down the aisle with my dad by my side. It all seemed surreal. I wasn't supposed to have the fairy-tale dream, I still had cancer! I remember wondering what all the guests thought. I was sure someone out there was thinking something dark, especially during the "to comfort and nurture, in sickness and in health, until death parts you" section. But it didn't matter. It was magical. We vowed to be fellow adventurers, willing to continually grow beyond self-imposed limits, and to keep alive curiosity and humor no matter what life threw us.

Our vows said it best: "You marry a mystery, an other, a counterpart. In a sense the person you have married is a stranger about whom you have a magnificent hunch. This person is someone you love, but his depths, her intimate intricacies, you will come to know only in the long unraveling of time."

In my case my diagnosis *made* my marriage, but in other cases it can break one. Like it or not, your cancer experience will reveal the depth of your partner's potential. When the going gets tough, will he be a valuable team player or will he just bail? When I say bail, I don't just mean physically leave you. A partner can vacate while he or she is still sharing your bed (and probably stealing the blankets!).

Checking out emotionally is not an option.

It's important to be open and honest and to communicate. Silence helps no one. Give your partner a chance to understand you. It's quite possible that he'll be more supportive than you think. If not, remember this: "Your rejection is God's protection." Give him the boot and walk on, Sista, walk on. Too many women feel trapped once they get sick. They're afraid to be alone and afraid to start over. But the stress and sorrow caused by a partner who is permanently out to lunch just aren't worth it. You've already been through way too much to be saddled with a deadbeat!

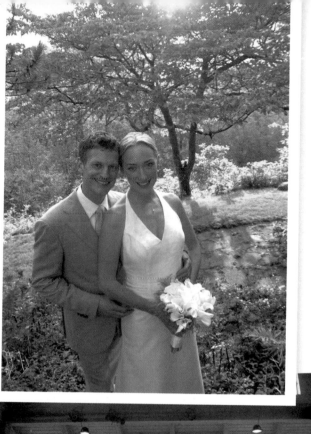

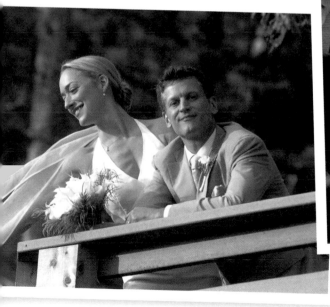

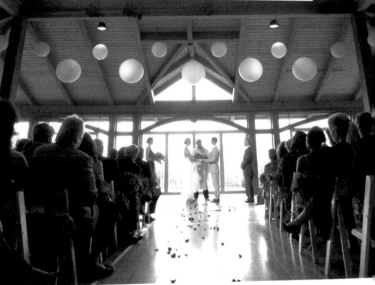

PROFILE:
LINDSAY NOHR BECK

AGE: 30

HAIR COLOR: Brown

EYES: Green

HEIGHT: 5'7"

WEIGHT: Are you kidding? Not fair, I just had a baby!

HOMETOWN: New York City

OCCUPATION: Founder and executive director of Fertile Hope

FAVORITE SAYING: "Life is what happens when you are busy planning it."

BEST TIP: Live the life you always imagined.

lindsay's icon:

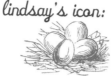

tip no.72

"YOU GOT TO BE IN IT *to win it!*"

How can you win the lottery if you don't buy a ticket? Don't wait until everything is back to normal and just right before you scratch and win. Go out with friends and get involved in social activities. Mr. or Ms. Right will not show up on your doorstep. Find a support group for people your age dealing with the same issues as you and talk about what overwhelms you and what your goals are. Or check out sites like www.CisforCupid.com. No need to wonder if a potential mate will "get" you, all participants on this dating site are cancer survivors! Remember the power of fire-engine-red lipstick on the mirror. Manifest your man! He is out there. Start your witches brew!

Lindsay:

At age twenty-two I was diagnosed with tongue cancer and was treated with aggressive radiation therapy. At twenty-four it returned, spreading to my lymph nodes. My second treatment regime included surgery, chemotherapy, and a second round of radiation. After having radiation twice to my head and neck area, I don't have a ton of saliva. A few months after dating Jordan, my now husband, I went to one of my standard checkups, and my doctor commented that my saliva production had increased dramatically and asked if I knew why. With a huge smile on my face, I answered, "I have a boyfriend." He looked at me funny. What in the world could that have to do with saliva? Then it hit him, and we both started giggling uncontrollably. Of all the things they told me to do to improve saliva production, kissing wasn't on the list!

After having one-third of my tongue removed, not to mention being a two-time cancer survivor who might be infertile, dating was scary. My mind was flooded with questions: When someone kissed me, would he notice that part of my tongue was missing? Should I tell him in advance or just go for it? Who would want me? If the tables were turned, would I want me? Part of me resented the fact that boys could judge and or reject me based on things that might happen to them one day (one in two people will get cancer in their lifetime!) and that they didn't even know about themselves (for instance, they might reject me because of infertility when they didn't know their own sperm count). As a result, I was picky, if only as a means of self-preservation. For two and a half years, I didn't really date. I think part of me wanted to and part of me didn't. It didn't help that I was introduced to boys as: "Lindsay, my friend who had cancer"! My sex life was nonexistent for about three years.

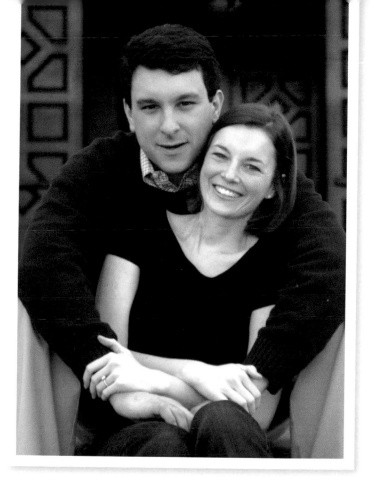

Then I met Jordan, and we got busy making up for lost time! I remember telling him it had been awhile and that he would be my "first since cancer." He looked shocked. How do you respond to that? I also asked if he'd been tested for STDs and HIV—a question I always thought should be asked, but I'd always been too chicken to bring it up. Now it seemed extra important—no boy was worth more medical drama.

(P.S.: My husband swears he can't tell that my tongue is any different!)

EXPLORE SOME CANCER
kama sutra

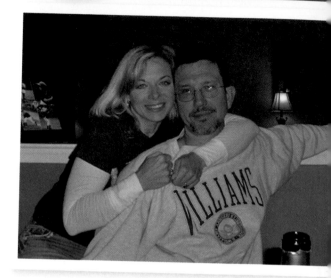

Dare to be lusciously lip-smackin! Don't shelve yourself or your erotic sparks. We may not be able to control our lives but we can control how we respond to them, especially when it comes to sex.

Sexuality is a natural part of being human. When we're ashamed of it or have an unhealthy connection to it, we squash a zesty piece of ourselves.

If you're not ready to be with a lover, be your own. There is a divine spark flowing through your feminine splendor. What better way to stay in touch than to stay in touch (so to speak)? Baths, candles, oils, pretty lingerie—it's called goddess worship, ladies!

As I write this I have to laugh. I've returned all the beautiful lingerie I got for my wedding, I sleep in ratty boxers, I fly around like a maniac who refuses to soak in the calming waters (though I own a hot tub), I hate to cuddle—*That's your side, this is mine, and my legs are so dry right now that my skin is peeling off in sheets!* I could really stand to listen to my own advice. My husband would probably appreciate it, too. It's sometimes hard to remember the goddess within, but a little reverence is like vegan chicken soup for the soul.

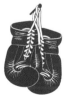

Terri:

Sex is unbelievably life affirming anytime, but especially when you are plagued with thoughts about your own mortality, sex can banish fear and make you feel alive. Good sex during treatment makes you feel normal. Radiation and body scans can make you feel like a lab rat, but sex with a hot, loving partner made me feel like me. It was a reminder that life goes on, a respite from decisions and scary thoughts. It wasn't just sex that made me feel that way. Slow body massages, foot massages, a back tickle session (you know, the light-touch kind) were all things that made me not only feel loved, but still powerful, myself, normal.

If your partner treats you like you're broken, it makes you feel broken. As women we feel the need to take care of everything and everyone. But when I was being treated, I needed Vic (my husband) to hold my hand, quiet my fear, and at the same time treat me normally, which included having as much sex or more than usual—just because it felt good.

Even if you don't feel like sex, or if being intimate with another just isn't part of your current equation, adore yourself. Do you own a vibrator or some playful toys? If not, invest and educate. If parts of your anatomy have changed, explore them. Hell, even if they haven't, start snooping around. How can you feel comfortable letting someone else touch you if you can't quite stomach it yourself? Your acceptance is the most important step you can take toward a healthy sexual life. Keep an open mind and think of it as important self-tutelage. Most of us grew up in a house where sex talk was taboo and uncivilized. Unpack that baggage and explore some bondage!

tip no.74

TAKE THE *tour*

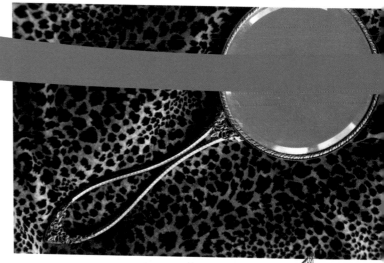

After Terri sent me the above entry, we had a hilarious cell phone conversation. Ever hear of Dr. Betty Dodson? The infamous sex educator and international authority on women's sexuality? Dodson is the mother of masturbation and has been teaching women how to love, nurture, and get off while holding a hand mirror for decades. Terri and I call it "taking the tour." Of course while we were yammering about this subject, I was stuck in an elevator full of straitlaced corporate types. Though I tried to whisper, as soon as someone mentions sex everyone in earshot develops bionic hearing. I wonder how many of those nine-to-fivers reached for the hand mirror when they got home.

Terri:

After being diagnosed I was reading tons of books on cancer and health and being a woman. I was also searching for grounding and something to help soften the fear of my own mortality that I was desperately trying to avoid. So I stumbled upon an article in an empowering woman's mag that made a correlation between having a poor sense of direction and being ignorant about your vagina. Since I have always been extremely directionally challenged, I embraced this article as the answer to my problems. I would, in earnest, explore the nether regions of my own anatomy, and I was certain this would give me the answers I sought. What an excellent distraction from radiation!

I bought a beautiful hand mirror and some scented candles, cranked up a Barry White CD, and made a date to go exploring. Something about learning about my body, taking time, being kind, and loving myself sexually on purpose had an incredible effect on me. It reinforced

181

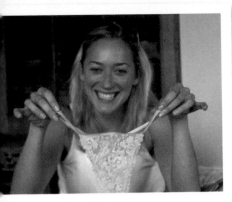

that I was a woman, a sexual being very much alive and totally committed to staying that way.

When you have had a cancer diagnosis, no matter how many people love you, there are moments when the alone nature of this journey becomes undeniable.

Creating a real relationship with yourself, sexual and otherwise, is a true gift to glean from your experience.

The postscript on my internal GPS adventure is that the last time I tried to take the E to 53rd and Seventh, I ended up in Queens and thought I was in Hoboken! But I know exactly where my labia majora is.

tip no.75

SAY PLEASE AND THANK YOU,
but ask for what you want!

Whether you romance alone or with a partner, sex is very healing, especially when it's done with a higher consciousness. Tune into your private late-night, smooth-moves radio station. Don't zone out! Pay attention and respond to what feels good. If you're in a relationship, remember that your partner isn't psychic. This is not the time to shut down and say things like "I don't know" and "nothing" when you're asked, "What's wrong?"

Grab your sexual megaphone, speak up, and be specific.

Remember, too, that it isn't all about you! What? Scandalous! Your partner has needs, too, and sometimes you have to serve it up to keep it coming. Deliver the goods even if it's just a quick FedEx. I hear hospital sex can be quite a turn-on.

Not that intimacy is just about messing around. It isn't. Holding hands, love pats, hair brushing, cuddling on the couch, long walks, or just sitting in quiet peace and reading together can be delectable. Heart-to-hearts are purifying. The power of the words you use and the depth of the conversations you explore can jack intimacy up to a whole new and divine level.

CRAZY SEX CANCER FACTOIDS

- Believe it or not, some patients have seen a dramatic increase in their red blood cells post-orgasm. So peek under those covers and have some fun!
- Wilkes University in Pennsylvania says that individuals who have sex once or twice a week show 30 percent higher levels of an antibody called immunoglobulin A, which is known to boost the immune system.

Planet Cancer holds year-round retreats for young people with cancer. In 2007 they held the first-ever couples retreat in the country! If these retreats are anything like Heidi, prepare to have a blast and open up your can of cancer whoop-ass!

Heidi:

I knew there was a need for a venue for young couples (cancer survivors and their co-survivors) to reach out for support. I went through my own treatment as a single gal, for the most part. (My boyfriend at the time broke up with me four months into treatment. My mother would still throttle him on sight if she saw him.) So while I was concerned about my immediate family members and their emotional needs, I could selfishly put myself at the center of my treatment universe without a second thought. The couples at our retreat, on the other hand, were each primarily—and quite selflessly—concerned about the other's well-being.

We had two separate discussion groups, one for the patients and one for the "cancer partners" (a new term that we coined over the weekend). Many of the issues that they brought up separately were the same: How to share raw emotions while protecting the other. How

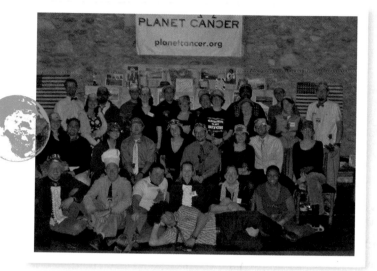

to adjust to a new normal. How to give up/take on responsibility. How to deal with friends and family members as a team. How to handle kids. How to recognize changes in personality and the relationship caused by the disease and treatment, and how to redefine the relationship accordingly.

The underlying issues seemed to be the challenge of being honest without burdening each other. And, conversely, how each could be selfish at times without feeling guilty or as though it was at the expense of the other. I think everyone realized that it was okay, and even necessary at times, for each to put themselves first: Cancer partners needed to take care of themselves in order to take the best care of their patient, and patients needed to put themselves first to give their treatment the maximum chance for success.

I have always known that there were few outlets for younger adults in their twenties and thirties with cancer (thus the creation of Planet Cancer), but there are even fewer places for their partners to reach out for support as individuals, and no place at all for couples to reach out as a team. I felt that the weekend was a success because it allowed partners to meet other folks in the same boat,

and to have a safe place to experience and express difficult emotions without being judged. And also because they all got to spend a weekend as a couple surrounded by other couples who just got it. They didn't have to constantly give their backstory.

{ children CAN be part of your future }

It's hard to believe I'm not twenty-five anymore, and I don't have all the (fertility) time in the world to figure out just when I want a little Jack or Jill. Couple that with cancer and bam! I've always wanted kids, yet the thought of bringing them into my cancer world is so frickin' scary. I don't plan on having this disease forever (no matter what my wonderful doctors say), but I have it for now, and now is when the clock is ticking. Talk about a conundrum. More than likely the stable cancer that is in my body wouldn't affect my pregnancy. But no one knows for sure whether the hormone shifts a pregnancy would cause in my body could wake the sleeping dragon. I guess it's something my husband and I will have to research more about. We'll have to dig deep to figure out whether or not it's a risk we're willing to take.

Making a decision to have a child is yours and yours alone. Of course your partner has a huge say, but ultimately you have the final word, especially if it involves your body. And be prepared for everyone to weigh in. Some people may even criticize you, dishing out a how-could-you sort of scolding. Just take the best and leave the rest. No one else can walk in your high heels.

Many women are not told that cancer treatments can cause infertility and premature menopause until it's too late.

Unfortunately, many oncologists don't think beyond your survival. They don't worry about you moving on with your life. I guess in their book, just being alive is good enough. And while it is, it's still important for you to have

FERTILE HOPE

I met my posse gal Lindsay when I started to explore other fertility options for young women with cancer. There aren't many epithelioid hemangioendothelioma babes with babes out there, so it seemed impossible for me to connect. In fact, Dr. Demetri said I might be the first to try. I doubt that's true but, oh, how reassuring! If you're one of those babes, give me a shout-out. I would love to hear how you're doing.

Fertile Hope, Lindsay's organization, is a national, non-profit group dedicated to providing reproductive information, support, and hope for cancer survivors. It seeks to educate women about the fertility issues they face. It also offers a program called Sharing Hope, which gives financial assistance for and increased access to procedures and treatments for men and women diagnosed with cancer in their reproductive years.

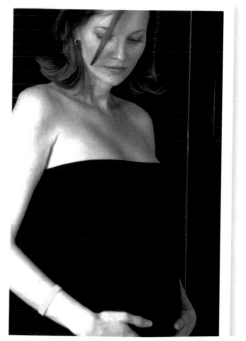

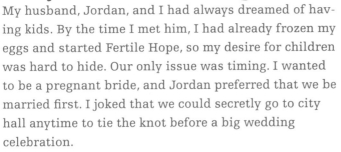

Lindsay:

My husband, Jordan, and I had always dreamed of having kids. By the time I met him, I had already frozen my eggs and started Fertile Hope, so my desire for children was hard to hide. Our only issue was timing. I wanted to be a pregnant bride, and Jordan preferred that we be married first. I joked that we could secretly go to city hall anytime to tie the knot before a big wedding celebration.

In the end we waited until our honeymoon to start trying. Our path to parenthood was full of ironic twists. After several miscarriages and three in vitro fertilization cycles, our dreams came true. We now have a nine-month-old little girl, Paisley Jane, and she is the light of our lives. Not only does she bring us unimaginable joy, but she is our legacy. As cancer survivor and co-survivor, there is a certain comfort in knowing that no matter what happens to us, we will live on through her.

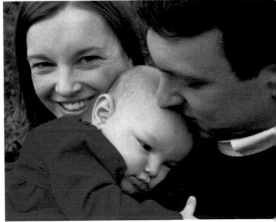

the option to have a family. It's a crime to take that option from you needlessly. Remember, you're the CEO of Save My Ass Technologies, Inc. When it comes to family planning, do your homework and be informed.

The good news is that more options exist than ever before. Fertility preservation and parenthood after cancer are definitely possible.

Most importantly, know your risks, know your fertility status, and know your options.

Little-known fact: Whether or not you get your period back after cancer treatments, if those treatments damaged your reproductive system, you will go into menopause early. Timely family planning is key!

tip no. 76

EDUCATE YOURSELF,
on your options

When I asked Lindsay what advice she would give a dear friend who was newly diagnosed with cancer, she emphatically responded, "Freeze your eggs, now!" Point taken. Whether you choose to follow that suggestion or not, there are many options for starting that family you always dreamed of. Lindsay provides much more information on her Web site, www.fertilehope.org, but here's an edited overview:

surrogacy

If you're unable to carry a pregnancy, you might turn to a surrogate, a woman who will carry your baby for you. In some cases a family member or friend acts as a surrogate; you can also find one through an agency or a clinic. Traditional surrogacy involves using the male partner's sperm to inseminate the surrogate. Gestational surrogacy means that a couple creates an embryo through in vitro fertilization; the baby is then transferred to the surrogate for gestation.

assisted reproductive technologies (ART)

Assisted reproductive technologies is a broad term that refers to achieving pregnancy by artificial or partially artificial means. It includes taking medications to induce ovulation as well as the use of egg or embryo donors.

If you can't use your own eggs—but can sustain a pregnancy—donor eggs or embryos might be an option. Eggs are retrieved from a donor, fertilized with the male partner's sperm, and transferred to your uterus. You'll receive hormone support as long as needed.

Embryo donation, on the other hand, is a new alternative that allows a couple to experience pregnancy and birth together, though neither of you will be genetically related to your child. Most commonly, embryo donors come from another couple undergoing ART. Excess embryos are frequently frozen; if a couple chooses not to use them, they may donate them. It's less common to create embryos strictly from donor eggs and donor sperm.

adoption

It is possible to adopt if you've had cancer, but you should know that many agencies use your medical history as one of their criteria. In addition, many foreign countries have their own specific requirements for potential parents' health. It's important to choose an agency and country that are open to working with cancer survivors.

The average cost of adopting a child in the United States varies according to the type of placement, but it can range from nothing (if you're adopting a child from the foster care system) to more than $30,000. It may also take a long, long time for the arrangements to be finalized—often it's more than five years before new parents can take their child home.

tip no. 77

DON'T FORGET YOUR
youngest co-survivors

"**If they could just** stay little 'til their Carter's wear out." Remember that slogan? Well, they do grow up no matter how you wish you could just stop time at the moment they're the cutest and you're a goddess.

When you have cancer, you're not the only person who's scared— kids need understanding and kindness even when you don't feel up to it.

They need knowledge, too, and getting the information directly from you is best. Kids will wonder what cancer is, why people get it, if they will get it, and if you'll be cured. Whether they say so or not, they will worry, and trying to shield them isn't always the wisest course of action.

Being honest with your family, including the youngest members, can provide a sense of safety even if the information they hear is hard to swallow. Remember the monsters under the bed? Kids have vivid imaginations. Let them

know that both you and your doctor are doing everything possible to help you get well. Also, your kids' teachers and the other adults in their life should be aware of what your child is going through, and be prepared to offer added support.

Do be ready for the possible cancer tantrums. That's right: They get to pull 'em, too! Regression, clinginess, confusion, and intense fear are common. When these tantrums go down, cover your kids with blankets of your love and let them know how much you adore them.

Terri:

My husband Vic's first wife died of cancer when she was twenty-nine, leaving him to raise three young children, who were five, three, and one at the time. Twelve years later the two of us fell in love—six months before my diagnosis. He was and is a total rock star. He went to every doctor's appointment with me and took care of me emotionally by staying positive. He also treated me normally, which was important.

The boys had suffered such a huge loss in their lives that they seemed nonchalant about it all. Alex, our fifteen-year-old middle son, actually said to me over sushi after my diagnosis: "Like if this thing is terminal, it's not like I am going to sit in my room and cry about it."

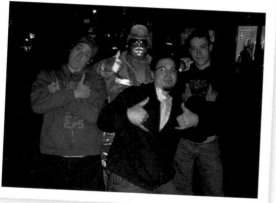
Terri's boys

Ouch! Kids say the darndest things! But I maintained my composure and said, "Given your background I understand how you could feel that way, but you know what I am sure of is that I love you and I'm not going anywhere now or ever!" But after the exchange, I went home and cried privately in my bedroom even though I knew he was just scared and a teenager and mad at the possibility of losing another mother.

Terri's story shows how important it is to let your kids process the information in their own way. Be prepared for them to need their own dose of attention. It's also crucial to have your spiel prepared before you speak to them. Every kid will react differently—there is no right or wrong way to respond to the news. Some will break down; others will want to broadcast the story to the world for comfort and attention.

Suzanne:

The day I was diagnosed, I left work early to go see my thirteen-year-old daughter Sophie play soccer. I had promised Sophie I would tell her what was going on even if it was bad. I had to keep my promise.

Her team won the game four to two, very exciting, but what I was not looking forward to was the car ride home. I told Sophie the news in the back of our Volvo. Tears streamed down her face as we

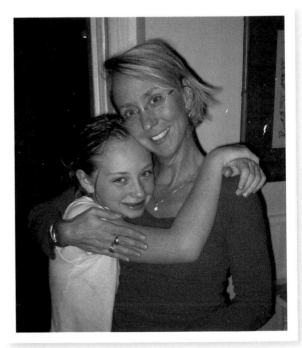
Suzanne and Sophie

held hands in the backseat. I didn't even understand what was going on, so how could I expect her to grasp the situation? We talked a lot that night, and I made her look at me a lot. I kept saying: "Look at me, I am super-healthy, and I promise you I am going to beat this." I don't know if she believed me, but she seemed a bit at peace, so I let her get on instant messaging and tell her boyfriend and some of her other friends about it.

I had to give Miss Mermaid (her nickname) room for her feelings. The first thing she wanted to do was tell the world. Thankfully I am a very open person. My daughter loves a little drama and loves the attention so the way for her to deal with it was to get sympathy from her friends and pull her own version of the Cancer Card at school. I have never seen a kid get out of so much homework! But it was okay—it was her way of coping. We just had to put a lid on it all by alerting her teachers and getting her some professional help. So after chemo it was off to the kid shrink! After her therapy sessions we'd talk all about it.

One poignant moment was the third day of my chemo. It was pouring rain. Steve wasn't able to be with me, and I just started crying over my cereal. I didn't want to go that day. Yuck. Rain, cancer, who needs it! My despair flipped Sophie out a bit, but I believe she needed to see that it wasn't all easy for me. Even though I went to work after chemo every day like a robot, it wasn't easy. Seeing me struggle gave her some much-needed perspective.

chapter eight in review:

remember:

Get creative with your new body. Try something new to please it.

Love and affection with the right person can help you feel more normal and nurture a healing that goes beyond your cancer baggage.

Cancer can ignite an inner revolution and sexual liberation—if you let it.

Be straightforward and communicate. Give your partner a chance to understand and support you.

If you're thinking about starting a family, do your research. There are more options now than ever before!

Remember, your cancer affects your kids, too. They need understanding and kindness even when you don't feel up to it.

You are an amazing woman whose needs and desires deserve to be met!

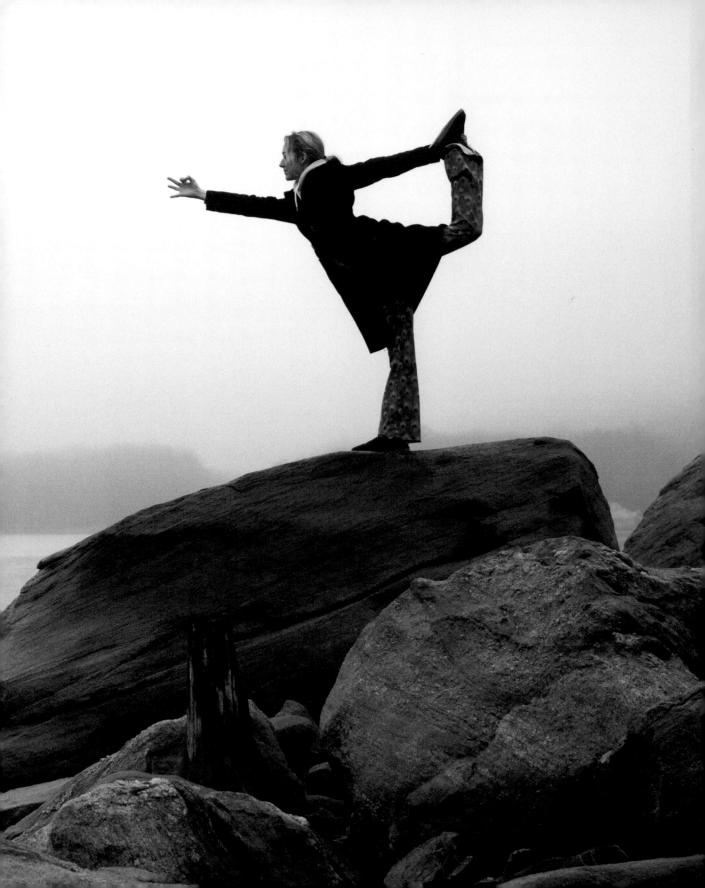

conclusion

By completing this book you have officially graduated from Cancer Babe to Cancer Cowgirl. Yee haw! Cancer Cowgirls are a divine order, a free-spirited bunch of powerful women who take charge as they gallop through life's obstacle course. We don't whisper, we ROAR! This is just the beginning, a match to the tinder of curiosity, possibility, and tenacity we all possess. You are complete now. You are whole now. For God's sake, you're a Cancer Cowgirl! A heavenly creature full of sass and fireworks. A dazzling warrior full of peace and fury.

Cancer Cowgirls past and present are survivors. Take the best and leave the rest. Don't forget to feel the ground beneath you and notice the groovy scene as you hitchhike down the highway of one-day-at-a-time. Remember, too, that you are not alone. Your posse is waiting for you. Connect, share, and pen your own tips. Stay in touch! I miss you already. Send me your stories, faux pas, hijinks, and advice: Info@crazysexycancer.com.

Peace, veggies, and a lot of glitter,

kris

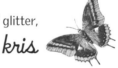

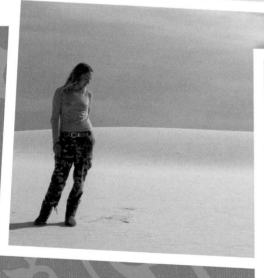

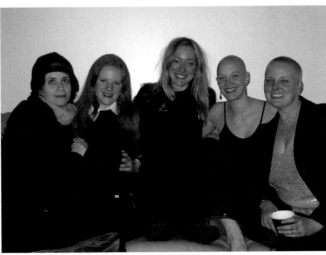

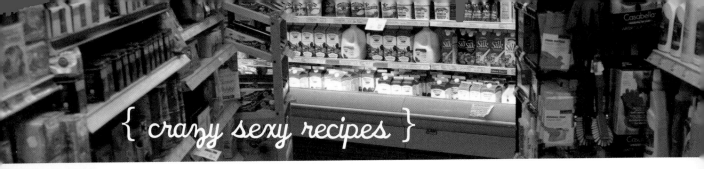

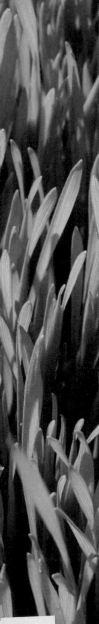

When I was a little girl, my grandma used to cut and collect recipes, storing them in a metal index box. That box was her prize possession, all her secrets locked inside. Today it belongs to me. I still have all her recipes—in fact, I've revamped quite a few—but I've also made room for my own.

I want to encourage you to think outside the box, too. Don't be afraid to stray and experiment. I never follow the rules. Measurements are guidelines to me. Basically I just write down what I need and then toss it all together, seasoning to taste. The result: a dish catered to my palate. Remember, choose organic whenever possible. Here are just a few of my standards to get you going.

nectar of the goddess

I make this every morning without fail! This juice is the secret to good health, abundant energy, and overall glow.

Cucumber (I like to juice 2 for sweeter nectar)

Celery

Broccoli stalks

Sweet pea sprouts, sunflower sprouts, or both

Kale

Throw all the ingredients into the juicer and get ready to zoom.

lemon crush

Divine lemonade, but don't let it sit around or the stevia will get bitter.

1 peeled lemon (sans pits)

ice

water

2 scoops of stevia

Once again, throw everything in the blender and go! Add a Fuji apple for a super treat and mint for a booze-free julep.

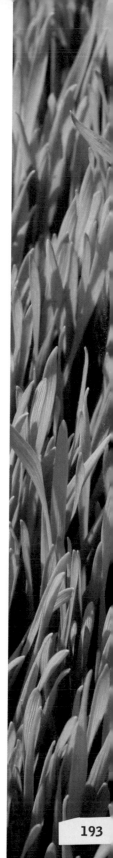

key lime smoothie

Avocado

Peeled and seeded lime

Coconut water

Cucumber

Stevia

Toss everything into a blender, whir, and enjoy. You can also add some shredded dry coconut as a garnish, or different alcohol-free flavored extracts. Try the Frontier or Simply Organic brands. Add some raw cacao and peppermint extract and you've got a tasty peppermint patty.

peace salad

I call this Peace Salad because it includes every color of the rainbow—and therefore loads of enzymes, chlorophyll, phytonutrients, vitamins, and minerals. Yum!

Use any of the following or add what you like. Just make sure the result is colorful.

Organic mixed greens: romaine, arugula, or spinach

Cucumbers

Red peppers

Carrots

Broccoli florets

Diced red onions

Shredded purple cabbage

Any sprout (my favorites are sunflower and mung bean sprouts)

Avocado

Shredded jicama

Oil-cured olives

bliss bruschetta

Chopped red onions

Garlic

Parsley

Basil

Tomatoes

Celtic Sea Salt

Combine all the ingredients and spread on sprouted bread like Ezekiel brand. (Sesame is the best. You can also buy raw breads online.) This goes great with a big salad.

a.l.t.

This is a hearty sandwich, good for an easy lunch or travel.

Avocado

Romaine lettuce

Alfala sprouts

Celtic Sea Salt

Sprouted bread

Organic mustard

You can use one of the pesto dressings (see following pages) as a spread, or try the Mock Mayo!

sacred sweet potatoes

Slice sweet potatoes into ¼-inch rounds and spread them out on a baking sheet. Drizzle with tahini and chopped fresh rosemary. Bake for about 20–25 minutes. Add Celtic Sea Salt to taste.

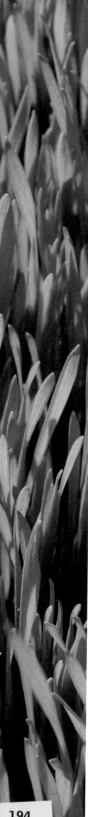

TWO-MINUTE DRESSINGS AND SPREADS

Because you don't have time to dillydally! Make these condiments with a whisk or throw them in the blender. I have a little mini Cuisinart that's great for one or two servings of dressing. Easy to use and fast to clean.

sexy vegan caesar dressing

Tahini

Olive oil

Flax oil

Water

Yellow miso

Dulse flakes

Garlic

This concoction can be slightly heavy, so use the water to thin it out. I generally use the oils in equal proportions, and add one spoon each of miso and tahini. Miso is pretty salty, though, so you might like less. Also, I love garlic (it's a natural antibiotic, blood thinner, and cleanser), so I use two cloves, but look out, mama! One clove should do it for most people.

hippieville house dressing
A Woodstock standard.

Olive oil

Flax oil

Garlic (of course)

Celtic Sea Salt or nama shoyu

Fresh-squeezed lemon

Pinch of cayenne or Spice Hunter Zip (love this condiment)

avocado dill dressing

You'll definitely need the blender for this one. You can also add a touch of olive oil to make it creamier.

Avocado

Fresh dill

Garlic

Celtic Sea Salt

Water

Scallions

mock mayo

Several cups of macadamia, cashew, or pine nuts

Lemon

Celtic Sea Salt

Dry or stone-ground mustard

Turmeric (just a dash or two)

Paprika

Blend all the ingredients. If it's too thick, add a splash of filtered water.

electric lotus pesto

It's so easy! You can use spinach or basil and either pine nuts, macadamia nuts, or walnuts—basically whatever you can get your hot little hands on. If an ingredient isn't available, improvise! Pesto can be used over pasta or as a spread for a sandwich or wrap. Thin it with a little water and you've got a dressing.

Version one:

Basil

Macadamia nuts

Garlic

Extra-virgin olive oil

Lime juice

Celtic Sea Salt

Version two:

Spinach

Cilantro

Walnuts

Lemon

Extra-virgin olive oil—or splurge and try hemp seed oil (yum)

Garlic

prana sauce

Pretend you're Italian and don't measure; just throw the stuff in the blender and taste.

Lots of little yellow tomatoes or grape tomatoes. Add some plum or vine-ripe tomatoes, too. Basically, you're looking for sweet ones. Get extra because people usually prefer more sauce.

A few bunches of basil leaves

Sea salt to taste

Garlic cloves

Prana means "life force," and this sauce is alive and kickin'!

resources

GREAT SHOPPING SITES

Here's where to buy those sassy, in-your-face cancer T-shirts, plus other cool cancer must-haves. My favorite shirt du jour reads MY ONCOLOGIST IS MY HOMEBOY.

- www.cafepress.com
- www.cancersucks.com
- www.chemochicks.com
- www.gotcancer.org
- www.planetcancer.org. Heidi Adams's site offers shopping and more. In my opinion the g-string is a showstopper!

POSSE BLOGS, WEB SITES, ORGANIZATIONS, AND INFO

- www.baldisbeautiful.org. Sharon Blynn's Web site. Bald Is Beautiful seeks to provide inspiration to women dealing with the physical and mental challenges of cancer. The site shares tips on how to feel gorgeous on the outside and inside!
- http://cancervixen.com. A delicious graphic novel about battling cancer by Marisa Acocella Marchetto. It's very *Sex and the City* meets cancer!
- www.crazysexycancer.com. Moi! You'll find more resources, handy information, recipes, tips, and Cancer Cowgirl stories. Check in from time to time and look for posse workshops, boot camps (wicked fun, not hard or exhausting), and wellness weekends near you. Let's create a national stitch-and-bitch!
- www.fertilehope.org. Lindsay Nohr Beck's organization. This site offers information about all the options available to a Cancer Cowgirl who wants to start a family. More than just a checklist of options, the site offers honest, nitty-gritty details that will help you make the choice that's best for you.

- www.glamour.com/lifestyle/blogs/editor. Erin Zammett Ruddy's blog. Follow the day-to-day experiences of this "Red hot mama." Erin chronicles the many ups and downs of surviving cancer.
- http://jackiefarry.com. Visit Jackie's site and stay informed about her latest rockin' projects and escapades.
- www.liveforthechallenge.com. Diem Brown's foundation. On this site you can set up your very own gift registry. It's sort of like a wedding gift registry, only instead of china and blenders, you list stuff that will help you in your fight for your health! Your family, friends, or even strangers can then go on the site and purchase an item from your list, like groceries, maid service, a wig, a plane ticket, or even a nice spa treatment!
- www.nylifelab.org. Jodi Sax's organization. The LifeLab is an organization for cancer survivors working to figure out what they want to do with their lives post-diagnosis. If you've decided that a major life or career change is in order and you happen to be a New York City gal, this is the place for you. Also check out the writing program. Remember, creativity heals.
- www.planetcancer.org. Heidi Adams's foundation. This is a fun and fabulous community site for young adults with cancer. It's a place to share insights, hash over fears, or even give the finger to cancer with folks who understand exactly where you're coming from. Check in whenever you can—Heidi will keep you informed of all the cool (and important) events going on in the young adult cancer community.
- www.terricole.com. Check out Terri's therapy/life coaching and Reikki work. She's my kick-ass mentor!
- http://therackpack.org. Allison Briggs's organization. The Rack Pack is a generous organization dedicated to helping young cancer gals make ends meet.

MORE AWESOME SITES FOR YOUNG ADULTS WITH CANCER

- **http://berniesiegelmd.com** and **www.ecap-online.org.** These two Web sites by Dr. Bernie Siegel offer a wealth of resources, information, and tools based on the science of mind-body-spirit medicine.

- **www.cancerandcareers.org.** This kick-butt site has tons of tools for the survival kit. It's a great resource for all women with cancer, not just the ones hustling home the bacon. Browse away—it'll really help you become proactive and organized. You name it, this site covers it—from how to wash your wig to how to apply for disability.

- **www.cancercare.org.** I love what this organization writes about its services, so I'm not gonna try and jazz it up (most sites are so dry): "CancerCare is like a professional cancer assistant, answering your questions, finding you help, or just listening when you need an understanding ear." It even has resource links for cowgirls with rare cancers like mine. Love it! Here's another perk: If you can't afford a wig, these folks will provide one to you for free.

- **www.cancersurvivorsunite.org.** Camps and support programs for young adults with cancer.

- **www.cisforcupid.com.** An online dating site for cancer survivors!

- **www.gildasclub.org.** Gilda's Club (named for Gilda Radner) provides places for men, women, and children living with cancer—and their family and friends—to come together and build social and emotional support—free of charge.

- **http://heardsupport.org.** This site is specifically designed for peeps with my type of unique (and yes, special) cancer. HEARD informs and unites Hemangioendothelioma patients so they can share, compare, comfort, and assist each other, as well as present a strong and combined group to make people aware of this cancer.

- **www.lef.org.** The Life Extension Foundation has been introducing life-saving medical discoveries and funding scientific research for more than 25 years.

- **www.livestrong.org.** Everything about this site is geared toward a winning attitude. It's Lance Armstrong, for God's sake! Check out the resource section and look for the organizational binder. Navigate your way to the Livestrong Young Adult Alliance section, too. The organization's mission is to improve survival rates and quality of life for young adults living with cancer by promoting research, generating awareness, and providing these survivors with a voice.

- **www.plwc.org.** People Living with Cancer is a patient information Web site of the American Society of Clinical Oncology (ASCO). This site provides oncologist-approved information to help you make informed decisions about your health care.

- **www.pregnantwithcancer.org.** Need I say more? Yes! This organization can connect a newly diagnosed pregnant goddess with a veteran pregnant goddess who has gone through a similar cancer with a bun in the oven. Share your experience and get support.

- **www.raibenefit.org.** Rise Above It provides grants and scholarships for cancer survivors.

- **www.shopwellwithyou.org.** A great site for women to find guidance on how to use clothing and accessories (my favorite form of therapy) to maintain a positive body image during and after treatment. There's advice on everything from swimsuits, pocketed bras, and skin care to lymphedema and ostomy garments. Go shopping!

- **www.stepsforliving.org.** A "social resource portal" that uses the power of the arts to raise awareness about what it means to be a cancer survivor by educating and empowering young adults.

- **www.ulmanfund.org.** This cool site provides support programs, education, and resources—free of charge—to benefit young folks and their families and friends who are affected by cancer, and to promote awareness and cancer prevention. Check out Doug and Diana Ulman's book, *No Way, It Can't Be!: A Guidebook for Young Adults Facing Cancer.*

- **www.vitaloptions.org.** Probably the most complete list of resources I have come across! This is one-stop-shopping. Plus, every week its creator Selma Schimmel (a pioneer in the young adult movement) hosts a radio show called *The Group Room*. To find out more, browse away.
- **www.youngcancerspouses.org.** This organization is dedicated to bringing together young spouses with cancer to share information, stories, support, and advice. Check out the forum—a great way to connect with other couples experiencing the ups and downs of the cancer roller coaster.

BEAUTIFUL YOU

- *Beauty Therapy: The Ultimate Guide to Looking and Feeling Great While Living with Cancer* by Ramy Gafni. This book will help you continue to look your most beautiful while you're fighting your cancer battle. From wigs to makeup, skin care, and developing your own beauty rituals, this guide has it all!

STYLISH HOSPITAL GOWNS

- **www.lazygirldesigns.com.** Download your own fabulous hospital gown pattern and get crafty.
- **www.spirited-sisters.com.** Dignified and super-classy hospital garb. I'd wear these robes to work if I didn't work for myself!

WIGALICIOUS STUFF

The best place to start when it comes to getting info about wigs is your stylist. These pros usually know the top local spots for faux follicles. In addition to CancerCare, call the American Cancer Society for more information. Many shopping malls and department stores have fun wig shops, too. Also, Google your wig ideas—lots of sites come up for sexy pink numbers!

- **www.locksoflove.org.** If you're not going to use your locks for your own wig, donate them to a child in need.

- **www.wigsalon.com.** A huge selection of fun and fashionable wigs.
- **www.wigsite.com.** Lori's Wigsite is an education, to say the least.
- **www.heavenlyhats.com.** This site offers free hats for anyone with a medical need!

INSURANCE STUFF

These sites will help clear up the inevitable insurance questions and dilemmas that you'll face:

- **www.healthinsuranceinfo.net**
- **www.patientadvocate.org**
- **www.patient.cancerconsultants.com**

DISABILITY INFO

Some good Web sites with helpful information on disability benefits:

- **http://cancerguide.org/disability.html**
- **www.thedisabilityexpert.com/**
- **www.ssa.gov/applyfordisability/**

TRAVEL FOR CANCER PATIENTS

- **http://aircharitynetwork.org**
- **www.cancerpatienttravel.org.** Offers charitable travel and housing arrangements.
- **SkyWish** through Delta Air Lines. (800) UWA-2757, ext. 285.

BREAST CANCER

- **www.asklisacole.com.** Lisa's an expert at helping women find the bra that works for them post-lumpectomy or -mastectomy.
- **www.breastcancer.org.** Offers a ton of information about breast cancer.
- **www.cancer101.org.** Get organized with this site's awesome binder! You'll also find valuable information to help you navigate your way through your diagnosis.
- **www.lookgoodfeelbetter.org.** Look Good . . . Feel Better hosts seminars and offers support to folks dealing with the many physical issues that arise when fighting cancer.

- **www.mdanderson.org/diseases/Breast Cancer.** Besides being one of the best cancer hospitals in the world, M. D. Anderson's site offers a lot of information and advice on breast reconstruction.
- **www.plasticsurgery.org.** A service that provides background on the history and wide variety of cosmetic and reconstructive plastic surgery procedures as well as offering a plastic surgeon referral service.
- **www.self.com.** Check out *Self* magazine's breast cancer handbook from October 2006.
- **www.sistersnetworkinc.org.** This organization is committed to raising awareness of the impact that breast cancer has in the African-American community.
- **www.y-me.org.** If you're fighting breast cancer and feeling alone, check out this site, which will connect you with another breast cancer goddess like yourself.
- **www.youngsurvival.org.** An international nonprofit network of breast cancer survivors and supporters dedicated to the concerns and issues that are unique to young women with breast cancer. Through action, advocacy, and awareness, the Young Survival Coalition seeks to educate the medical, research, breast cancer, and legislative communities and to persuade them to address breast cancer in women forty and under. It also serves as a point of contact for young women living with breast cancer.

EAT YOUR VEGGIES, SHAKE YOUR ASS STUFF

retreat centers

These centers can guide you through detox and lifestyle upgrades:

- http://annwigmore.org
- www.hippocratesinst.org
- www.livingfoodsinstitute.com. Brenda Cobb's institute.
- http://optimumhealth.org
- www.treeoflife.nu

alternative health updates and news

- **www.mercola.com.** An awesome alternative medicine resource and education site.

supplements, treats, books, appliances, and info

- www.hippocratesinst.org
- www.highvibe.com
- www.live-live.com
- www.rawfood.com

jump!

- **www.needak-rebounders.com.** Mini trampolines!

cleaning out the pipes

- **To find a colon therapist** trained in the gravity method (the most recommended style), check out the Colon Therapists Network at www.colonhealth.net/therapist-search.
- **For enemas,** look for Fleet or Cara enema bags, both usually available at your local pharmacy.

a few appliances to get you started

- **My favorite juicer** is the Green Star (www.greenstar.com). It extracts the most juice and also allows you to make pâtés, nut butter, cracker batter—even banana ice cream or sorbet!
- **For travel and/or wheatgrass,** I use my trusty hand-crank juicer. You can find one at www.healthyjuicer.com.
- **The Cadillac of blenders** is the Vita-Mix. This blender has made my life so much easier. Visit www.vitamix.com or order through some of the sites already mentioned.
- **Don't forget** your Cuisinart (www.cuisinart.com)!

READING LIST

- *A Cancer Battle Plan: Six Strategies for Beating Cancer, from a Recovered "Hopeless Case"* by Anne E. Frähm with David J. Frähm

- *The China Study: The Most Comprehensive Study of Nutrition Ever Conducted and the Startling Implications for Diet, Weight Loss and Long-Term Health* by Dr. T. Colin Campbell with Thomas M. Campbell II

- *The Cure: Heal Your Body, Save Your Life* by Dr. Timothy Brantley

- *Diet for a New America: How Your Food Choices Affect Your Health, Happiness and the Future of Life on Earth* by John Robbins

- *Eating in the Raw: A Beginner's Guide to Getting Slimmer, Feeling Healthier, and Looking Younger the Raw-Food Way* by Carol Alt

- *Everyday Grace: Having Hope, Finding Forgiveness, and Making Miracles* by Marianne Williamson

- *Living Foods for Optimum Health: Staying Healthy in an Unhealthy World* by Dr. Brian R. Clement with Theresa Foy Digeronimo

- *Love, Medicine and Miracles* by Bernie S. Siegel, MD

- *The pH Miracle: Balance Your Diet, Reclaim Your Health* by Dr. Robert Young

- *The Raw Food Detox Diet: The Five-Step Plan for Vibrant Health and Maximum Weight Loss* by Natalia Rose

- *Raw Food Real World: 100 Recipes to Get the Glow* by Matthew Kenney and Sarma Melngailis

- *The Raw Gourmet* by Nomi Shannon

- *A Return to Love: Reflections on the Principles of a Course in Miracles* by Marianne Williamson

- *Spiritual Nutrition and the Rainbow Diet* by Dr. Gabriel Cousens

- *The Sunfood Diet Success System* by David Wolfe

- *The Wheatgrass Book: How to Grow and Use Wheatgrass to Maximize Your Health and Vitality* by Ann Wigmore

{ acknowledgments }

Oceans of love and thanks to all the people who added feathers to the wings of this book; especially to Scott Watrous for his fearlessness and insight, Nikki Hardin for her warrior Goddess trailblazing, and my brilliant editors Mary Norris (my newly appointed godmother and queen of the ever alluring fridge magnets), and hot mama Imee Curiel for her wit and sword-like pen. To Bonnie Bauman for her additional shaping, emotional bourbon, and sweet fire. To Karen Kelly for giving me technicolor training wheels. To my pistol-packin' agent Maura Teitelbaum, get out of her way now! Thank you for believing in me. Your YES changed my life. To Beth Blickers, the original angel, you rock! To the dazzling Inger Forland for sisterhood soul powwows and big dreams, and to Justin Loeber for all his jazz and razzamataz.

Endless gratitude and deep bows to the divine broads who make up my sensational posse, especially Erin Zammett Ruddy (Red), the graceful Lindsay Beck, and my wild child Heidi Adams. Big love to Marissa Ronca (you are a genius and a truck driver) and all the amazing folks at TLC (especially Brooke Runnette and Don Halcombe) for starting the Crazy Sexy Revolution. To Dave Marsh for always encouraging me to kick ass and challenge people. To my dear friend Lisa Cocciardi for her tireless support, shoulder, and beautiful photography (especially the radiant and soulful cover shot). May we find New Mexico again. To all the other uber-talented artists and photographers who contributed their work to this book, especially Big Daddy Andre Costantini. To the sassy and soulful Karla Baker for capturing my personality in her creative designs. To Sheryl Crow and Pam Wertheimer for their big hearts and generosity. A divine thank you to Marianne Williamson for taking me under her electric wing. To Donna Karan for encouraging me to find the calm in the chaos while still being stylish. Unconditional love and endless thanks to my family (Aura, Leslie, and Doppler Dad Ken) for letting me air our laundry and encouraging me to cliff dive nude. To my rock solid cowboy husband Brian for his deep love, support, and excellent edits—you're next buddy! Finally, thanks to all my teachers and gurus for inspiring me to question the box and think outside of it.

PHOTO / ART CREDITS

All photographs are by Kris Carr except for the following:

Spot art throughout provided by ClipArt.com, IndexOpen.com, Photos.com

p. iii by Lisa Cocciardi

p. iv Peace Hands by Lisa Cocciardi & Kris Carr

p. 2 Sheryl Crow by Sheryl Nields

p. 8 Kris "a frickin' mess" by David Zellerford

p. 18 Kris Carr by Brian Fassett; Allison Briggs courtesy Allison Briggs; Diem Brown courtesy Diem Brown; Erin Zammett Ruddy by Basil Childers; Heidi Adams by Elena Dorfman; Jackie Farry by James Sevigny; Jodi Sax courtesy Jodi Sax; Lindsay Beck by Michelle Walker Photography; Marisa Acocella Marchetto by Jeremy Balderson; Cancer Vixen icon courtesy Marisa Acocella Marchetto; Melissa Gonzalez by Karen Pearson/MergeLeft Reps; Sharon Blynn by Greg Kessler; Suzanne Donaldson by Richard Imrie; Terri Cole by Eric Stephen Jacobs

p. 24 Kris on tracks by Lisa Cocciardi

p. 26 Kris in curlers by Brian Fassett

p. 29 Kris & grandma by Andre Costantini; Kris headshot by Chia Messina

p. 33 Erin by Basil Childers

p. 37 Kris on lawn chair by David Zellerford

p. 43 Kris with cancer books by Brian Fassett

p. 45 Kris on plane by Brian Fassett

p. 49 Terri by Eric Stephen Jacobs

p. 52 Leslie by August Goulet

p. 58 Kris in car by David Zellerford

p. 62 Suzanne by Richard Imrie; Suzanne in chemo chair courtesy Suzanne Donaldson

p. 63 Heidi by Elena Dorfman

p. 64 Heidi and Lance Armstrong/Heidi and twins courtesy Heidi Adams

p. 73 Kris on trapeze by August Goulet

p. 75 Marisa Acocella Marchetto by Jeremy Balderson

p. 76 Marisa in sunglasses courtesy of Marisa Acocella Marchetto

p. 78 Jodi courtesy Jodi Sax

p. 80 Erin & Kris by Brian Fassett

p. 84 Kris at monastery by Lisa Cocciardi

p. 86 Kris with tea by Lisa Cocciardi

p. 90 Kris & Bhagavan Das by Brian Fassett

p. 91 Marisa courtesy Marisa Acocella Marchetto

p. 96 Kris/Brian birthday cake by Aura Carr

p. 109 Kris & Diem by Brian Fassett

p. 111 Kris with sign by Brian Fassett

p. 113 Jackie and Cindy courtesy Jackie Farry

p. 115 Melissa by Karen Pearson/MergeLeft Reps; Little Erin & Melissa courtesy the Zammett family; adult Erin and Melissa by Karen Pearson/MergeLeft Reps

p. 116 Melissa in chemo chair; Melissa, Andrew, and Erin by Dan Hallman

p. 117 Melissa and Andrew courtesy Melissa Gonzalez; Allison courtesy Allison Briggs

p. 119 Allison with friends courtesy Allison Briggs

p. 120 Allison courtesy Allison Briggs

p. 121 Oni by Arthur Cohen courtesy Oni Faida Lampley; Oni at computer by Brian Fassett

p. 122 contact sheet by Andre Costantini

p. 145 Brenda Cobb by Jane Holmes

p. 154 Kris with glasses by Aura Carr; Sharon Blynn by Robin Emtage

p. 155 all photos courtesy Sharon Blynn

p. 157 Diem courtesy of Diem Brown

p. 158 Diem by Lorenzo; Diem and friends courtesy Diem Brown

p. 159 Jackie by Brian Fassett

p. 160 Melissa photos by Karen Pearson/ MergeLeft Reps

p. 165 Lisa Cole courtesy Lisa Cole

p. 166 Ramy by Mike Falco courtesy Ramy Gafni

p. 177 Kris & Brian wedding photos by Andre Costantini

pp. 178 and 179 Lindsay Beck photos by Michelle Walker Photography

p. 180 Terri and Vic courtesy Terri Cole

p. 183 Planet Cancer retreat courtesy Heidi Adams

p. 185 Lindsay courtesy Lindsay Beck; Lindsay, Jordan, and Paisley by Michelle Walker Photography

p. 188 Terri's boys courtesy Terri Cole

p. 190 Kris yoga by Brian Fassett

p. 191 posse by Brian Fassett

p. 191 and p. 201 Kris desert by Lisa Cocciardi

Type set in Egyptienne (Adrian Frutiger), Bell Gothic (Chauncey H. Griffith), Griffith Gothic (Chauncey H. Griffith and Tobias Frere-Jones), and Varsity Script (Jason Walcott), Letter Gothic (Roger Roberson), CG Behemoth (Dave West) and Engravers (Robert Wiebking)

Photoshop Brushes and Diesel Font from Misprintedtype.com

Finally!
A skirt that fits!
skirt!magazine.

www.skirt.com